Fundamental Aspects of Palliat

Note

Health and social care practice and knowledge are constantly changing and developing as new research and treatments, changes in procedures, drugs and equipment become available.

The authors, editor and publishers have, as far as is possible, taken care to confirm that the information complies with the latest standards of practice and legislation.

Fundamental Aspects of Palliative Care Nursing

An evidence-based handbook for student nurses

Second edition

Robert Becker

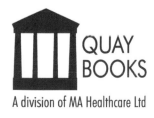

QUAY
BOOKS

A division of MA Healthcare Ltd

Quay Books Division, MA Healthcare Ltd, St Jude's Church, Dulwich Road, London
SE24 0PB

British Library Cataloguing-in-Publication Data
A catalogue record is available for this book

© MA Healthcare Limited 2010

ISBN-10: 1 85642 394 8
ISBN-13: 978 1 85642 394 6

Printed by CLE, Huntingdon, Cambridgeshire

Foreword

Wow! What a roller coaster of emotions this book has evoked. I am really pleased to find out that the reactions I had to death and dying are in fact quite normal. The chapter on bereavement also highlighted and finally put a context to one event that I'll always remember. After my mother died, people I had known all my life seemed to ignore me. I realise now it was because they didn't know what to say, but at the time it's the feeling of isolation that takes a long time to fade. There was also the time I offered a hysterical lady a cup of tea while she was running around the Chapel of Rest. After reading the chapter on communication skills I realise that it was not a completely insensitive thing to say. (This was something that happened in my first year as a student and on my very first placement.)

The book is very user friendly; the text is academic, but written in uncomplicated English, which I found very helpful as I have a form of dyslexia which makes reading difficult at times. It gives an excellent insight into palliative care, and the self- assessment tests are an absolute must so that you can test your understanding of a topic. The three parts help a lot by grouping things together and the chapter headings make it easy to find areas of interest.

For me the book is an excellent survival guide for nursing students with regard to the difficult area of palliative care. Every student knows that death and dying are things that we encounter throughout our three years of training and I really wish I had had this book at the beginning of my training to help guide me through. I will definitely be recommending it to other students and I hope it makes it onto university reading lists.

Deanna Tompkins
Nursing Student, Staffordshire University

As a student nurse entering my final year of study I was honoured to be asked to write this foreword. It is imperative in my view that end of life care is done compassionately and correctly. It is something that we as student nurses do not look forward to confronting, but will inevitably do so many times during our training and nursing career. It is something we want to do well and something we are petrified of getting wrong. This book guides, advises and supports us through these very difficult times and teaches us ways in which we can do all the right things, answer the difficult questions and provide the best possible care for every dying person we encounter. The book also expresses perfectly the importance of this through the medium of the short story to paint a picture at the beginning of each chapter from the perspective of the person who is dying.

The user-friendly style of this handbook enabled me to navigate easily towards any specific area of palliative care I required. The overall format and content not only create a clear guide for student nurses, but also include sections which enhance self-learning, including the 'Reflective activity' and 'Self-assessment test' segments in each chapter. I found the use of different symbols throughout the book very handy to easily locate these exercises.

The reflective activities helped me to build confidence in my clinical practice, by asking me what I would do in certain scenarios. This helped me to visualise situations and to think carefully about how I would handle them. I also found that this was a trigger for reflection on my personal experiences in the clinical placements I have attended to date. I will definitely feel more at ease and in control when confronting similar situations in the future and I will certainly utilise this informative and useful handbook throughout the remainder of my training and take it with me into my nursing career. A great book.

Abigail White
Nursing Student, Staffordshire University

Contents

Contents

Preface

It is now five years since the first edition of this book was published and whilst the core skills and behaviours required to care for the dying in multiple environments have remained constant, the knowledge base to support this care has developed and changed in some important areas. It is appropriate therefore that this second edition takes a fresh look at the new evidence- and practice-based experience that has become available to inform care in this dynamic area.

The primary focus of the book is now on student nurses, who have many competing demands during their education, but are consistently exposed to palliative care scenarios throughout their three-year training and find such care emotionally exhausting and academically challenging. I also know that they care very much about getting it right, and whilst there are numerous high-quality books on the market that are available to support academic study in this area, this book is currently the only one specifically designed for their learning needs in everyday clinical practice.

Rather than providing a detailed meta-analysis of theoretical and research-based concepts, the emphasis in the text is on dealing with practice-based situations in a sensitive and informed way. This second edition is therefore designed to be a compact, learning-oriented, evidence-based handbook which offers comprehensive, practice guidelines across the spectrum of palliative/end of life care scenarios to provide a trigger and opportunity for reflection and learning.

I have taken the opportunity to redesign the layout of the chapters to make them more structured and user friendly by the use of symbols to help the reader easily locate the relevant information they need. I have also included some educationally important elements, such as learning outcomes at the outset of each chapter to guide the reader, reflective points and activities to help with professional development, and self-assessment multiple choice tests at the conclusion of each chapter to consolidate learning. There is even a true or false quiz offered for those who would like to test their knowledge before or after their studies. The short clinical anecdotes at the outset of each chapter which served well to set the scene in the first edition have been retained and changed only where necessary.

I have also added several new chapters to help readers make sense of the range of new initiatives that have come to the fore in palliative care in the last five years. Even the language has changed and we now hear the term 'end of life care' used in many contexts where 'palliative' was used before. Essentially they are one and the same, but government strategy and policy documents have introduced this phrase for a good reason. The term 'palliative', whilst generic in its meaning and intent, has nevertheless become synonymous with hospices, specialisation and above all cancer. There is a real need to find a term that is clearly understood by the general public and embraces caring for the dying of whatever diagnosis in whatever environment. 'End of life care' does just that and signals an intent to meet everyone's needs.

Overall, the integrity of the text remains fundamentally the same. It was the intention with the first edition to produce a book that was very much an evidence-based 'how to do it' text, and feedback from many sources (including the formal reviews), confirmed that this was a successful and much appreciated approach. It is with this in mind that the focus was moved towards student nurses and their learning needs. Post-registration learning opportunities in palliative care abound in the UK for qualified nurses, with a proliferation of study courses available in both the higher education sector and local hospices. Some are tied to academic pathways, while others offer a more flexible online or distance learning approach. Each has its merits and the growth of such educational opportunity has undoubtedly contributed greatly to the high degree of skills employed by nurses in many sectors of healthcare where end of life issues are of importance.

Pre-registration nursing curricula are constantly developing alongside service developments to reflect the need for nurses to be well prepared for the demands of clinical practice in many environments. The learning needs in a palliative context of the next generation of nurses have, however, been systematically ignored by successive statutory bodies. There remains to this day no formal imperative to include any specific end of life care content in the pre-registration nursing curricula on any part of the nursing register. Consequently, provision ranges from the fully integrated and structured module through to the odd lecture given by a local clinical nurse specialist if they can spare the time and have the skills. This is simply not good enough. As any competent educator will confirm, if you can inform, inspire and shape attitudes, skills and behaviours at the outset of a career, then nurses will carry this learning with them throughout their working lives. The potential therefore to empower the role models of the future is enormous, and whilst crowded curricula and complex politics may preclude more formal inclusion of palliative care knowledge in the short term, it is hoped that in some small way this text will fill a much needed gap in the market and provide students of nursing with a user-friendly but challenging reference book that will help them in both their studies and – more importantly – at the bedside of those who die in multiple environments across the healthcare system.

The Nursing and Midwifery Council of the UK published a new edition of their Code of Professional Conduct in 2008, so the links to appropriate clauses that are relevant to chapter content have been updated accordingly. It is now more important than ever for nurses to be able to utilise the code to support care, so that they can assure themselves of delivering best practice at all times.

Internet content in palliative care has exploded in the last five years and there are now many more highly professional websites that offer a wide range of information for nurses to access to guide practice. The difficulty, however, is knowing which ones are of decent quality. Not all are regularly updated and many have a dual role to provide important information to patients and families as well as to health professionals. Successfully finding your way to one that may prove useful can be a time-consuming and frustrating exercise. Those included in the text have been reviewed carefully for ease of navigation and quality of content.

Some years ago, on a humanitarian aid teaching visit to Russia, I was struggling in the classroom to find the words to express the essence of palliative care and used a simple analogy to get the message across. I likened it to a blend of the head, hands and the heart, the most important of which is the heart. It's a common analogy to which I make no claim, but in the context of the moment it worked well with my Russian audience and has worked well ever since when I've used it in a number of other countries, as well as in the UK. Finding the right words to articulate the real meaning of the palliative approach is not easy, but it's important that we do, so that when challenged to justify our actions in the hard-pressed culture of care we work in we can make a convincing argument that stands up to ethical, financial and humanitarian scrutiny. The argument works both ways of course, and the real test of any civilised society is not only how it deals with the funding and promotion of good health for its citizens, but also how it funds and deals with those who are dying.

To have the opportunity to be at the bedside of someone throughout the final moments of their life is indeed a privilege for any carer. Few professions are allowed the honour of being part of this unique event in the way that nurses are and all of us have a vested interest in getting it right for our patients. One day it will be our loved ones and indeed ourselves who will be the recipients of such care and we would want it to be of the highest standard. This book will hopefully make a small, but significant contribution to helping to mould and shape the attitudes and skills of the nursing practitioners of the future, who may well be the ones at our bedside when a palliative approach beckons. I make no great claims for its efficacy, but I am confident that it can become a useful spanner in the toolbox of knowledge, skills and behaviours that nurses draw on in what is inevitably an emotive and sensitive life event.

Acknowledgements

Those of you familiar with the first edition of this book will notice immediately that one of the two original authors is missing from the credits. My colleague Richard Gamlin has taken the opportunity to retire from his position as Senior Lecturer Practitioner in Sunderland and has withdrawn from the production of this second edition. His contribution to the original authorship of this book was considerable and it is appropriate therefore that this is acknowledged. I wish him well in his retirement.

I would also like to acknowledge the support and encouragement given to me from a number of people while this second edition has taken shape. In particular I would like to thank my wife Christine for her wisdom and enduring patience and Maria at Quay Books for her support and enthusiasm. Also Deanna and Abigail for tasking time out from their busy schedules as students to write the foreword and last, but certainly not least, my trusted and vastly experienced education colleagues who were the critical friends with the manuscript when needed and helped enormously to keep me on track.

Palliative care quiz

Each of the 50 questions relates directly to material within the text of the book and the whole quiz will take you no more than 20 minutes to finish. Try completing the quiz before you read the book content to see how well you do. Keep a record of your score, and some time later, after you have attempted the reflective activities and the multiple choice questions at the end of each chapter, revisit the quiz. This will give you some idea of how much you've learned. You can also use this evidence within your professional portfolio to demonstrate learning.

		True	False
1.	Palliative care is only appropriate in situations where there is evidence of a downhill trajectory or deterioration		
2.	In palliative care, dying is seen as a normal life event		
3.	The practice of palliative care is compatible with aggressive curative treatment		
4.	The extent of the disease determines the method of pain treatment		
5.	To palliate means to relieve symptoms by the use of pharmacology		
6.	Hospice care is a concept and philosophy rather than a building		
7.	Given the choice most people would wish to die in a hospital setting		
8.	Competency assessment tools are an objective measure of job performance		
9.	Life closure skills, psychosocial care and teamwork are core areas of competency for nurses using the palliative approach		
10.	People dying in hospitals feel lonely and isolated from those around them		
11.	The provision of palliative care services requires emotional detachment		
12.	When encountering death for the first time it is useful to open the window afterwards to release the person's spirit and to bring fresh air around the bedside		
13.	Patient choice in how and where people die can be enhanced by the use of care pathways		
14.	The Liverpool Care Pathway and Gold Standards Framework have the potential to transform palliative care in the UK		

	True	False
15. Drug addiction is a major problem when morphine is used on a long-term basis for the management of pain		
16. Artificial hydration at the end of life can cause the patient more harm than good		
17. Advance directives (living wills) now have full legal status in the UK		
18. During the terminal stages of an illness, drugs that can cause respiratory depression are appropriate for the treatment of severe dyspnoea		
19. Individuals who are taking opioids should also follow a bowel regime		
20. Suffering and physical pain are synonymous		
21. Adjuvant therapies are important in managing pain		
22. The use of placebos is appropriate in the treatment of some types of pain		
23. In high doses, codeine causes more nausea and vomiting than morphine		
24. Morphine is the standard used to compare the analgesic effect of other opioids		
25. Managing symptoms other than pain is mostly about finding the right drug and dosage		
26. The pain threshold is lowered by anxiety or fatigue		
27. Manifestations of chronic pain are different to those of acute pain		
28. Pethidine is not an effective analgesic for the control of chronic pain		
29. Dyspnoea, nausea and constipation are the three most common symptoms reported after pain		
30. The very idea of an emergency in palliative care is a contradiction in itself		
31. Hypercalcaemia can be life threatening if not treated promptly		
32. Spinal cord compression appears rapidly and can resolve itself spontaneously		
33. Telling the patient the truth about their illness if they request it is likely to cause them harm		
34. It's always a good idea when handling sensitive questions to seek more information first from the patient		
35. Silences are difficult and are best handled by using open questioning		
36. The families feelings about the patient knowing their prognosis are always secondary to the patient's wishes		
37. Spiritual care is best delivered by those who know most about it, i.e. ministers of a faith		
38. Agnostics, atheists and humanists are people who can't make their mind up what they believe		

	True	False
39. If nurses are trained better to deliver spiritual care then it would make a big difference to the patients		
40. Essential comfort care around the bedside of the dying are mostly routine functional tasks that are better suited to a healthcare assistants role		
41. Last offices is a routine procedure that is best learnt from a policy manual		
42. During the last days of life, drowsiness associated with electrolyte imbalance may decrease the need for sedation		
43. It is crucial for family members to remain at the bedside until death occurs		
44. Cheyne–Stokes breathing is when the dying person's respiration becomes intermittent		
45. Natural light and normal conversation around the bedside of a dying person can help both patient and family		
46. Cultural care is full of sensitive pitfalls and it's best to call in faith leaders and let them deal with it		
47. Truth telling regarding diagnosis and prognosis varies in acceptability in some cultures		
48. Men generally reconcile their grief more quickly than women		
49. The loss of a distant contentious relationship is easier to resolve than one that is close or intimate		
50. Grief can best be described as a time-limiting process occurring through specific stages		
First score		
Second score		

PART I

Core concepts and developments in end of life care

This part of the book examines the central tenets that comprise the area of nursing we know as palliative care. It has moved a long way in the last decade and the skills that underpin how nurses can use the palliative approach are now much clearer and are examined here. Philosophical understanding of the concept of palliation as an active and dynamic approach has changed little, but this approach is now more systematically utilised by the UK government's End of Life Care Strategy and the development of care pathways. It is further informed by complex and important ethical debate which is constantly evolving and merits close attention. We also know that the drivers behind government strategy are aimed at meeting the needs of all those dying, of whatever diagnosis and in whatever environment; hence the need for a chapter which looks at some of the specific end of life care needs of the most common conditions encountered in clinical practice.

CHAPTER I

What is palliative care nursing?

Jenny was a strong, focused person in control of her life and illness. She came into hospital for pain control and we were able to sort that out quite quickly. She began to talk to me about her family, especially her husband, who had not come to terms with her terminal prognosis. Jenny felt she should be strong for him and not let him see her cry. I paused and said 'It's okay to cry you know'. She smiled, went silent for a while and the tears began to flow down her cheeks.

Learning outcomes

After reading this chapter and completing the reflective activities the learner will be able to:

- Define the terms 'nursing' and 'palliative'
- Understand how the concepts interrelate to each other
- Identify a range of core statements that characterise palliative care philosophy
- Relate key components of the various definitions of palliative care to nursing practice

Introduction

This chapter examines the diversity and challenges inherent in the nurse's contribution to palliative care. The art and science of caring for those who are dying and their families has long been recognised as an immensely demanding and rewarding part of health and social care. For nurses it is central to the values and principles that underpin clinical practice.

The science of palliative care has developed rapidly, due mostly to the central role of pharmacological interventions to help control chronic pain and distressing symptoms. This vital and essential aspect of optimising the patient's quality of life has undoubtedly contributed to the widening acceptance of palliative care as a recognised nursing speciality in the UK and beyond. The art of caring, however, has received significantly less attention, perhaps because of its more abstract nature. It is much more difficult to provide demonstrable clinical evidence of the successful contribution of interpersonal interventions to the overall quality of care to someone who is dying when the outcome is death itself. There is ample evidence, however, that a caring approach which embraces psychological, psychosocial and spiritual support is highly effective and is valued by both patients and families (Beaver *et al.*, 2000).

It can be argued that nursing and palliative care are natural partners in clinical practice and that the knowledge and skills learnt in this area are applicable to all nurses. People die in many environments and all have a right to supportive and palliative care regardless of diagnosis or circumstances (NICE, 2004). The particular knowledge, skills and attitudes needed to deliver quality palliative care will be explored in more detail in Chapter 2, but the values and beliefs that underpin such care are integral to good nursing. Nurses are in a unique situation, as the only real 24-hour carers in the healthcare system to incorporate and develop the principles and practice of the palliative approach into their daily practice where it is appropriate to do so. Therein lays both the paradox and the challenge to those nurses involved in end of life care: how to marry up the art and the science into a cohesive approach that reflects individuality, choices, dignity and compassion in whatever environment the care takes place.

Defining nursing

The activity of nursing is a complex mix of many hands-on skills and personal qualities bound together into an eclectic discipline that is inherently difficult to define. Florence Nightingale herself stated 'I use the word nursing for want of a better'. She went on to comment that 'the very elements of nursing are all but unknown' (Nightingale, 1860). Nursing is concerned with the human condition in times of health crisis and its very essence is therefore bound up in human nature.

The notion of professional caring, the building of therapeutic relationships and the practice of nursing as a regulated profession with definable standards has only been in existence since the beginning of the 20th century. In this time there have been many definitions of nursing published, but in the context of palliative care perhaps the most succinct and relevant one is that written by Virginia Henderson (1997):

> Nursing is primarily assisting the individual in the performance of those activities contributing to health and its recovery, or to a peaceful death.

The key phrases that stand out in this definition from a palliative viewpoint are 'assisting the individual... to a peaceful death'. The phrases suggest ideas of partnership, helping and dignity, all concepts that are central to the palliative approach to nursing.

Defining palliative

The word 'palliative' has its origins in the Latin word *pallium* meaning to cloak or cover, and in the context of how cancer was perceived and poorly diagnosed from the Middle Ages until perhaps the latter half of the 20th century, it is perhaps an appropriate description. Even today there are many cancers that grow unseen and without symptoms for some considerable time before the surrounding organs are affected and the person seeks help.

The notion of palliation is in itself very simple to understand. A more contemporary and simple definition is 'to mitigate the sufferings of the patient, not to effect a cure' (Macpherson, 2002). If we liken this definition to normal everyday ailments such as a head cold it becomes much clearer. There is currently no known cure for the virus which causes the common cold. Once a cold is contracted, the person experiences a range of symptoms over approximately 3–7 days and hopefully recovers. The experience is uncomfortable, but thankfully not life-threatening most of the time. The only relief obtainable is direct palliation of the most prominent symptoms, in the recognition that cure is not an option, but with the intention to improve our quality of daily life. As an experience it is one we can all relate to and in the context of end of life care the meaning is abundantly clear.

Current definitions

There are two key definitions to take into account. The WHO definition (Box 1.1) dates back to 1989 and was the first to define specialist palliative care. It was updated in 2002 and has been used by healthcare professionals and politicians worldwide to argue for the development of services and to guide practice in palliative care in over 100 countries (WHO 2009). It remains today the most accepted and used definition and the most challenging to those in developing countries where the medical model of care predominates. Take a look at the words and phrases in the definition and you will see why. The emphasis on quality of life and not quantity, the use of the term suffering, which can be both existential and physical and perhaps most of all the affirmation that dying is

Box 1.1 WHO definition of palliative care

Palliative care is an approach that improves the quality of life of patients and their families facing the problem associated with life-threatening illness, through the prevention and relief of suffering by means of early identification and impeccable assessment and treatment of pain and other problems, physical, psychosocial and spiritual
Palliative care:

- provides relief from pain and other distressing symptoms;
- affirms life and regards dying as a normal process;
- intends neither to hasten or postpone death;
- integrates the psychological and spiritual aspects of patient care;
- offers a support system to help patients live as actively as possible until death;
- offers a support system to help the family cope during the patient's illness and in their own bereavement;
- uses a team approach to address the needs of patients and their families, including bereavement counselling, if indicated;
- will enhance quality of life, and may also positively influence the course of illness;
- is applicable early in the course of illness, in conjunction with other therapies that are intended to prolong life, such as chemotherapy or radiation therapy, and includes those investigations needed to better understand and manage distressing clinical complications.

Ref: World Health Organization, http://www.who.int/cancer/palliative/definition/en/ Accessed: 15 April 2009.

a normal life process, not a medical disease process. Statements such as these still challenge us today, because they force us to think holistically and move away from a medical disease oriented model.

The key phrases and words that stand out from this definition are:

- quality of life of patients and their families
- the prevention and relief of suffering
- relief from pain and other distressing symptoms
- regards dying as a normal process
- neither to hasten or postpone death
- a team approach
- offers a support system... patient and family

The clear emphasis on support for both patient and family, combined with a multidisciplinary team approach, is consistent with good nursing practice and can help us to conceptualise what nurses should be attempting to achieve when they have contact with the dying. The definition can be criticised for mentioning treatments such as chemotherapy and radiotherapy, which implies that it is mostly applicable to cancer sufferers, however the primary statement at the beginning of the definition which mentions 'life-threatening illness' makes it clear that palliative care is for all diagnoses in whatever environment.

The National Council for Palliative Care, which is an umbrella organisation for setting standards in specialist palliative care in the UK, published its current definition in 2002 (Box 1.2). The main part of the definition is simply

Box 1.2 National Council for Palliative Care definition of palliative care

Palliative care is the active holistic care of patients with advanced, progressive illness. Management of pain and other symptoms and provision of psychological, social and spiritual support is paramount. The goal of palliative care is achievement of the best quality of life for patients and their families. Many aspects of palliative care are also applicable earlier in the course of the illness in conjunction with other treatments.
  Palliative care:

- Affirms life and regards dying as a normal process
- Provides relief from pain and other symptoms
- Integrates the psychological and spiritual aspects of patient care
- Offers a support system to help patients live as actively as possible until death
- Offers a support system to help the family cope during the patient's illness and in their own environment
- Supportive care is that which helps the patient and their family to cope with cancer and treatment of it – from pre-diagnosis, through the process of diagnosis and treatment, to cure, continuing illness or death and into bereavement. It helps the patient to maximise the benefits of treatment and to live as well as possible with the effects of the disease. It is given equal priority alongside diagnosis and treatment.

Ref: National Council for Hospice and Specialist Palliative Care Services. Definitions of Supportive and Palliative Care. Briefing paper 11. London: NCHSPCS. September 2002. Available to download at http://www.ncpc.org.uk/publications/archive.html

a shortened and adapted version of the one discussed earlier (WHO, 2009). What it significantly different, however, is the emphasis on the phrase 'supportive care', a term which is widely used today to describe both generalist and specialist services that may be required to support people at the end of life. It is based on an assumption that people have needs for supportive care from the time that their diagnosis is raised. The influential government strategy document on the development of palliative care services produced in 2004 by the National Institute for Clinical Excellence (NICE, 2004) uses this definition widely.

Once again we can see that the emphasis is on holism, support, dignity, choice and quality of life. Its real significance, however, lies in the influence of the consultation documents produced that preceded this definition and fed into the NICE Supportive and Palliative Care Guidance (NICE, 2004). Clear statements were made which talked about lessening future demands on the NHS and Social Services, the contribution palliative care makes to the health of the nation, and that it is an economic and compassionate response for a civilised society to adopt (NCHSPCS, 2000–2005).

Note that the concept of family is central to the wording of both these definitions and is repeated in a number of places. Many research studies have examined the complexities of family structure and dynamics and have rightly concluded that the cultural and societal influences, value systems and beliefs within a family will determine how they cope with major life crises such as death and dying (Andershed, 1999). What has become clear is that the 'family' is less well equipped in modern western society to deal with the emotional and social demands that caring for a dying relative brings than ever before (Johnston, 2004).

Palliative care services and professionals therefore have a real need to be flexible and non-judgemental in their interpretation of 'the family' and to be responsive to the changing norms of each community if they are to provide the support necessary to both the patient and those people important to them.

Palliative care nursing is very much about helping individuals to live until they die, and is not about helping them to die prematurely. This is not merely semantics, but a vital and integral part of palliative philosophy that is enshrined within the very simple statement 'neither to hasten nor postpone death' (Box 1.1) (WHO, 2009). Of all the components of this definition this is this one that is perhaps in danger of being undermined most. Both the Netherlands and Belgium have passed legislation in recent years to legalise medical assistance to die for those terminally ill people who request it. Switzerland also has legislation to enable individuals to request medical help to commit suicide and several states in the USA have similar laws. (Gordijn *et al.*, 2002)

There is no doubt that the intent behind such laws is indeed one of compassion for people who find themselves in a desperate situation. The euthanasia debate in its many complex forms will remain high on the healthcare agenda for many years to come. It is a sensitive issue than demands informed debate from all the healthcare professions. The moral prerogative in bedside care, however, usually falls on the nursing profession and it is useful to remember that with the correct use of the wide range of pharmacological interventions that are available today to control pain and symptoms, coupled with support for the family and patient, the statement 'help me to die', which is sometimes heard in this context, when explored carefully usually means 'help me'. Nurses who are aware of and embrace the palliative approach to care are able to do exactly that.

Using a range of disciplines and their expertise to address holistic needs is nothing new and has been a feature of modern healthcare for many years, yet few medical and nursing specialities have so fully embraced the idea as palliative care. Palliative nursing is guided by a belief in utilising such expertise at all levels for the benefit of the patient and family and makes a significant contribution to the enhancement of quality of life for people with a life threatening illness. Done well, it can be achieved in multiple environments and is not confined to the narrow corridors of specialism within a hospice setting.

Palliative nursing can make a difference

There are many genuine and heartfelt reasons why nurses find palliative care difficult, and most reflect the complexity and competing demands of caring for the dying in institutional environments and the home.

 Reflective activity

There are many reasons nurses cite for not being able to give adequate attention to the palliative care needs of their patients and the anecdotal comments below represent many of the heartfelt worries and concerns.

1. Scan down the list offered below and put a tick by the ones that are directly relevant to yourself and your work area.
2. Now revisit this list and narrow your choices with the following questions in mind:
    (a) Those things that are beyond my control and which I cannot change
    (b) Those things that I have some influence over and could possibly change
3. Now put together a short action plan based around those you have some influence over and set yourself a realistic time goal when you can review your success.

20 reasons why nurses find palliative care difficult

- We don't have enough staff where I work
- I don't have the time to deal with the complex issues involved
- There are too many other important priorities in my job
- I don't have the skills to deal with it
- I don't have the knowledge of drugs and symptom control
- I don't know what to say to patients and relatives why they ask difficult questions
- I'm afraid they might get upset
- I'm afraid I might get upset
- Getting upset means I can't do my job properly
- I haven't done a course on the subject yet
- I just find the whole business too much to deal with
- I'm afraid that I might get into trouble with senior staff if I spend too much time around the bedside and I haven't got a task to perform
- If something goes wrong, I'm afraid I might get the blame
- I've never had a major loss myself so how can I ever expect to understand and help someone who is dying
- This is just not the right place for someone to die, we don't have the specialists available
- The doctors try their best, but never seem to prescribe enough medication or tell people things in plain language
- We can never get a bed in the local hospice when we need one
- There's constant pressure to discharge patients early, which is inappropriate when you have dying patients on the ward
- I can't get the support I feel I need after a difficult death
- We can't seem to get the managers to recognise that death is something that happens frequently here, so there are no clear policies to deal with things

It would be all too easy to dismiss such reasons and to fall into the trap of the politically correct, who may cite developments in clinical governance, supervision, audit, staff appraisal, and the latest care management pathways as the answer to such anxieties. Whilst these developments have undoubtedly contributed to improved care and can empower staff in the right circumstances to push forward the agenda for the dying in their care, the daily reality for many clinical nursing staff remains overwhelmingly difficult.

This book could never present the reader with a universal panacea of answers for the issues that prevent the palliative care approach being utilised – indeed it would be arrogant to assume such – but it can and will challenge the reader to revisit the definitions and philosophies cited in this chapter and to review the merits of each as they use the good practice discussed within the text in their daily work.

Reflective point

Ask yourself about the care that you give in your everyday practice. Is it dominated by procedures, routines, assessments and practical tasks? (The science of caring.)

Or is it dominated by a more psychological approach, involving the use of counselling techniques and therapeutic work in groups or with individuals? (The art of caring.) Each is valid and we cannot expect to be skilled in all areas, but we can and should adopt a more balanced approach when the patient and family need it.

The End of Life Care Strategy

In the last decade there has been an ever increasing focus on patient choice and self-determination within health and social care settings. Within the UK there have been many initiatives (Commission for Health Improvement/Audit Commission, 2001; Department of Health, 2003; National Institute for Clinical Excellence, 2004) highlighting specifically that patient choice over place of death should be considered as one of the priorities for generalists and specialists alike, when caring for the dying.

The end of life care programme was set up in England in 2005 (NHS Confederation, 2005) to promote three initiatives which had been independently developed to facilitate good practice for dying patients: the Gold Standards Framework (GSF) (Thomas, 2003), the Liverpool Care Pathway (LCP) (Ellershaw and Wilkinson, 2003) and the Preferred Priorities of Care (PPC) document (Storey *et al.*, 2003). Three years after implementation, the Government's end of life care strategy (Department of Health, 2008) was published, which offers an ongoing evaluation of these three initiatives and their impact on direct care. Nurses in any environment where people die are now beginning to encounter these initiatives, which centre around planning and prioritising care for people in the weeks and months leading up to their death. The GSF is designed to be used by District Nurses and GPs and the LCP by all disciplines within acute care, long stay settings and nursing home environments, where it helps to prioritise care in the last week or so of life. The PPC, which is the only nurse-led initiative, is designed to be used with the patient to help plan and meet their wishes some months prior to their death in whatever environment.

 Reflective activity

Look around your workplace when you next have time and see if you can find a ward/unit/clinic philosophy of care. This is just a simple statement that recognises the orientation and priorities of care in your workplace. It may be kept in a filing cabinet somewhere, be with a student/staff induction package, or even on a notice board.

If there is one, read it carefully and ask yourself whether it embraces palliative nursing priorities and if there is a need to review the wording if it doesn't. If you work in an area where patients regularly die then this is important. If there is no statement of care philosophy then consider whether your workplace needs one and who to talk to so that you can help formulate one. In doing so, consider the palliative nursing priorities that may need to be included.

Conclusion

Embracing the palliative care approach successfully in nursing practice is not dependent on complex medical interventions, specialist environments, or even the instant availability of a range of drugs and disciplines. The propensity to specialise nursing as the preserve of the highly trained few does not apply here. The skills, attitudes and values that have been espoused in this chapter are applicable to nurses on any part of the register working in any environment wherever they encounter those dying of any diagnosis. Some of the most inspirational palliative care I have ever witnessed has been in situations where the building is riddled with damp, the floors infested with cockroaches and the modern opiates we take for granted to help manage chronic pain are simply not available. The suffering of the patient and family has been immense, but the skills of the nurses caring for them have been a privilege to see. It often that precious gift of 'being' and not just 'doing' alongside the patient which makes the difference (Thompson *et al.*, 2006).

Palliative care nursing involves valuing all the characteristics and past experience of the person. It demands an attitude and approach that goes beyond the diagnosis and immediate medical problem. Achieving this demands of the nurse a level of personal human contact with the dying person that goes beyond the tasks and procedures which can so often dominate everyday work. It is both a science and an art and emphasises normality and quality of life.

It values the whole person, and addresses their physical pain and discomfort, but also their feelings, their behaviours, their social issues and their family and friends. It is shaped by the individual's search for a sense of meaning and their desire for honesty, control over their life, and a need to maintain personal dignity, as they see it, for the life they have left. It is a combination of knowledge, skills and compassion in equal measure that is both sensitive, hopeful, meaningful and dynamic, but above all it is a way of thinking and an attitude of mind that should influence nurses' behaviour whenever they work with a dying person in whatever setting.

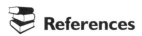

Reflective activity

It is often said that nurses make the worst patients, perhaps partly because they have a high level of knowledge and insight into the healthcare system they work in. Dying patients have expectations of that system and the care they want from nurses, but don't have the luxury of an insider view.

Take time out therefore and ask yourself: *If I were dying what would I want from the nurses caring for me?* Make a list of the qualities, values and attributes you would want from those caring for you. For example, you may wish to include: Being treated as a normal deserving patient and not ignored because you are a nurse and expected to cope.

When you have done this compare your list with the principles cited in the definitions and see how close your wishes are to the values espoused there.

References

Andershed, B. (1999) *The role of the family carer at the end of life: an evidence based literature review*. Swedish Board of Health and Welfare, Stockholm.

Beaver, K., Luker. K. and Woods, A. (2000) Primary care services received during terminal illness. *International Journal of Palliative Nursing*, **6**(5), 220–7.

Commission for Health Improvement/Audit Commission (2001) *National Service Framework Assessments No.1:NHS cancer care in England and Wales*. CHI/AC, London.

Department of Health (2003) *Building on the Best: Choice, Responsiveness and Equity in the NHS*. DoH, London.

Department of Health (2008) *End of Life Care Strategy. Promoting High Quality Care for All Adults at the End of Life*. DoH, London.

Ellershaw, J. and Wilkinson, S. (2003*) Care of the Dying. A Pathway to Excellence*. Oxford University Press, Oxford.

Gordijn, B., Crul, B. and Zylicz, Z. (2002) Euthanasia and physician assisted suicide. In: *The Ethics of Palliative Care: European Perspectives* (eds. D. Clark and H. Ten Have). Open University Press, Milton Keynes.

Henderson, V. (1997) *Basic Principles of Nursing Care*. International Council of Nurses, Geneva.

Johnston, G. (2004) Social death· the impact of protracted dying. In: *Palliative Care Nursing: Principles and Evidence for Practice* (eds. S. Payne, J. Seymour and C. Ingleton). Open University Press, Milton Keynes.

Macpherson, G. (ed.) (2002) *Black's Medical Dictionary*, 40th edn, p. 434. A. & C. Black, London.

National Council for Hospice and Specialist Palliative Care Services (2002) *Definitions of Supportive and Palliative Care*. Briefing paper 11. NCHSPCS, London. Available to download at http://www.ncpc.org.uk/publications/archive.html.

National Council for Hospice and Specialist Palliative Care Services (2002–2005) *Draft National Plan and Strategic Framework For Palliative Care*. NCHSPC, London.

National Institute for Clinical Excellence (2004) *Improving Supportive and Palliative Care for Adults with Cancer: The Manual*. NICE, London.

Nightingale, F. (1860) *Notes on Nursing: What It Is, and What It Is Not*, First American Edition. D. Appleton and Company.

NHS Confederation (2005) *Leading Edge, Improving End-of-Life Care*, Issue 12. NHS Confederation, London.

Storey, L., Pemberton, C., Howard, A. and O'Donnell, L. (2003) Place of death: Hobson's choice or patient choice? *Cancer Nursing Practice*, **2**(4), 33–8.

Thomas, K. (2003) *Caring for the Dying at Home; Companions on the Journey*. Radcliffe Medical Press, Oxford.

Thompson, G., McClement, S. and Daeninck, P. (2006) Nurses' perceptions of quality end of life care on an acute medical ward. *Journal of Advanced Nursing*, **53**(2), 169–77.

World Health Organization (2009) http://www.who.int/cancer/palliative/definition/en/. Accessed: 15 April 2009.

Original material for this chapter was taken and adapted from the following reference with full permission of the EMAP publishing group:

Becker, R. (2009) Palliative care 1: Principles of palliative care nursing and end of life care. *Nursing Times*, **105**(13), 14–16.

 Useful websites

The National Council for Palliative Care
http://www.ncpc.org.uk/

The World Health Organization
http://www.who.int/cancer/palliative/definition/en/

An exploration of the meaning of dignity in palliative care
http://www.ejpc.co.uk/ejpc/ejpc5no6.htm
http://www.acsu.buffalo.edu/~drstall/dignity.txt

Chapter links to the Nursing and Midwifery Council Standards of Conduct, Performance and Ethics for Nurses and Midwives (2008)

Section 1: Make the care of people your first concern, treating them as individuals and respecting their dignity

Treat people as individuals
■ You must treat people as individuals and respect their dignity

■ You must act as an advocate for those in your care, helping them to access relevant health and social care, information and support

Respect people's confidentiality

■ You must respect people's right to confidentiality

Collaborate with those in your care

■ You must listen to the people in your care and respond to their concerns and preferences
■ You must recognise and respect the contribution that people make to their own care and wellbeing

Ensure you gain consent

■ You must respect and support people's rights to accept or decline treatment and care
■ You must uphold people's rights to be fully involved in decisions about their care
■ You must be aware of the legislation regarding mental capacity, ensuring that people who lack capacity remain at the centre of decision making and are fully safeguarded

Section 2: Work with others to protect and promote the health and wellbeing of those in your care, their families and carers, and the wider community

Share information with your colleagues

■ You must keep your colleagues informed when you are sharing the care of others

Work effectively as part of a team

■ You must work cooperatively within teams and respect the skills, expertise and contributions of your colleagues
■ You must consult and take advice from colleagues when appropriate
■ You must make a referral to another practitioner when it is in the best interests of someone in your care

Section 3: Provide a high standard of practice and care at all times

Keep clear and accurate records

■ You must keep clear and accurate records of the discussions you have, the assessments you make, the treatment and medicines you give and how effective these have been
■ You must complete records as soon as possible after an event has occurred

■ You must ensure any entries you make in someone's paper records are clearly and legibly signed, dated and timed

☑ Self-assessment test

1. Palliative care philosophy is characterised by:
   A A medical model of disease control
   B Extending life and helping people to die
   C Supporting the patient and family through life-limiting illness
   D Admitting all the dying to hospices

2. In palliative care, dying is seen as:
   A A failure of medical treatment
   B A normal life event
   C A challenge to the multidisciplinary team
   D A rallying call for specialisation.

3. Which one of the following sets of words most accurately embraces Virginia Henderson's definition of nursing?
   A Dignity, teamwork and pharmacology
   B Partnership, helping and dignity
   C Self-respect, peaceful, and honour
   D Healing, personhood and partnership

4. Which of the following is the most accurate definition of 'to palliate'?
   A End suffering by curing
   B Relieve symptoms by use of pharmacology
   C Maximise quality of life
   D Relief of suffering recognising that cure is not possible

5. Which of the following sets of keywords most accurately describes the art of caring?
   A Relationships, closeness, presence
   B Professional, rational, efficient.
   C Organised, systematic, clear
   D Detached, clinical, observant

CHAPTER 2

Palliative nursing skills: what are they?

 'Will I ever be cured?' It is at times like this that we are faced with two simple choices. We can either 'go', make our excuses and change the subject, or 'grow', stay with the person and explore things further. On this occasion I chose to stay. He asked again if I knew whether he would be cured, but this time the intonation was different. It was as if he already knew the answer. I replied by saying to him that I knew very few details of his illness, but I would be happy to tell him what I knew, if that was what he wanted. He replied very positively, both verbally and with a nod of his head (Becker, 1999, p. 941).

Learning outcomes

After reading this chapter and completing the reflective activities the learner will be able to:

- Discuss the core knowledge, skills and attitudes required to meet the specific needs of patients and families in a palliative care scenario
- Relate the six core areas of palliative nursing identified to selected case studies
- Reflect on current skills and knowledge levels in the development of their own palliative nursing practice

Introduction

Caring for the needs of a dying person and those important to them is not only an important part of a nurse's role; it is also a formative life experience. The art and science of this encounter are embodied in palliative nursing. This chapter will explore the evidence base to support the diverse range of knowledge, attitudes and skills needed to provide nursing care for people at the end of their life.

Many nurses will have found themselves in situations similar to the one described in the short anecdote above and walked away wondering whether they acted correctly, said the right things and behaved with sufficient sensitivity to the dynamics of the moment. Later on they may have met with a colleague, their mentor or supervisor and told them the story of what happened, searching for some reliable affirmation that the skills used were appropriate and asking whether they could perhaps have done things any better. The reply they receive will depend very much on the experience, knowledge and wisdom of the person concerned and may range from the indifferent 'Well it sounds okay to me', through to a more counselling-oriented comment 'How do you feel about it now that you have had a chance to take stock?'.

Both these comments may be useful in some way, but equally they highlight the difficulty that nurses face in determining whether their competence to manage such delicate situations is sufficiently evidence-based or simply a combination of spontaneous intuitive responses based around life and work experience. The good news is that we now know quite clearly that good practice at the bedside in such situations has been shown to be a combination of both (Benner, 1984; Schon, 1987).

A close analysis of this encounter will elicit a whole range of skills that have been used to facilitate the conversation and it is important that we look at how these skills have been described in the literature to date. Doing so will give us a useful insight into the true nature of the diversity and essence of palliative nursing as it is delivered in clinical practice on a daily basis.

The evolution of competence in palliative nursing

Learning is a complex business and there are a number of ways to describe the way we attain competence in nursing, but for simplicity's sake an adapted version of Bloom's (1956) taxonomy, which emphasises individuals moving from a lower level of knowledge to a higher level of evaluation, can be used alongside a variation of Benner's (1984) 'novice to expert' thesis, which acknowledges critical thinking ability combined with technical skills. The work of Schon (1987) must also be considered principally because she recognised that it was the 'artistry' of practice which helped to differentiate between a competent and an expert practitioner, and as the clinical anecdote introducing this article illustrates, such artistry needs to be acknowledged.

This also relates very closely to Carper's (1978) four patterns of knowing which she suggests should be present in each nursing act, i.e. empirical knowledge, aesthetic knowledge, personal knowledge and ethical knowledge. Carper's work emphasises the influence of our values, beliefs and life experience in our work as nurses and has stood the test of time. There are elements of these four patterns observable in the current Nursing and Midwifery Council *Code of Conduct* (NMC, 2008).

The driving force towards developing competency assessment in both cancer and palliative nursing over the last decade has been the publication of a number of key documents. In 2002 the Royal College of Nursing (RCN) published their own Core Competency Framework for nurses working in specialist palliative care (RCN, 2002). This was the first time such a venture had been attempted and was useful in helping to clarify and define the role of nurses working beyond the hospice environment.

The National Core Competency Framework (RCN, 2003) attempted to pull together a uniform framework of standards for cancer nursing across four levels of practitioner and a wide range of skills. Many of the competency statements in this document were directly transferable to the palliative setting.

Both these documents have as their baseline premise the notion that competencies can best be assessed by the medium of observable behaviour in practice, backed up by a plethora of both written and verbal evidence. Higher Education Institutions (HEIs), however, find themselves (in the UK at least) with a proliferation of accredited courses for qualified staff at all levels that may be qualitatively excellent in the academic sense, but tend to concentrate on competency assessment via demonstrable critical thinking ability – and thereby lies the dilemma. How does nursing develop an acceptable model of competency assessment that embodies the best of both approaches?

In order to answer this we need to look a little further back in the literature. There are only a small range of authors who have attempted to define the skills and competencies used by nurses when caring for the dying (Davies and Oberle, 1990; Degner *et al.*, 1991; Heslin and Bramwell, 1989; Taylor *et al.*, 1997); see Table 2.1.

The work they have produced has been instrumental in helping others to develop working tools and frameworks to guide practice (Becker, 2000; De Vleiger *et al.*, 2004). See Table 2.2.

What is 'competency'?

There are numerous definitions available for the term *competency*, but we will concentrate on the definition cited by the RCN in relation to specialist palliative nursing (RCN, 2002, p. 2). Competence in a given set of skills can be defined as

> The skills, knowledge, experience, attributes and behaviours required by an individual in order to perform the job effectively.

Table 2.1 Core nursing skills for palliative care.

Davies and Oberle (1990)

1. **Valuing**: global and particular
2. **Connecting**: making the connection, sustaining the connection, breaking the connection
3. **Empowering**: facilitating, encouraging, defusing, mending, giving information
4. **Doing for**: taking charge, controlling pain, making arrangements, lending a hand
5. **Finding meaning**: focusing on living, acknowledging death
6. **Preserving own integrity**: looking inward, valuing self, acknowledging own reaction

Degner et al. (1991)

1. Responding during the death scene
2. Providing comfort
3. Responding to anger
4. Enhancing personal growth
5. Responding to colleagues
6. Enhancing the quality of life during dying
7. Responding to the family

Heslin and Bramwell (1989)

1. **Family care**: expression of emotion, enabling conflict resolution, teaching communication strategies
2. **Personhood**: as applied to both the patient and the nurse
3. **Symptom control**
4. **Life closure**: the totality of the death experience, before, during and after

In order to work therefore it relies on the formulation of agreed competency statements that are then identified at differing levels of practice.

At pre-registration level it is well established that it is the role of clinical staff to conduct practice-based assessments of competence. The issue of grading competency to practice in pre-registration programmes is straightforward. The assessor in the majority of instances is simply required to make a judgement, which indicates yes or no against a given statement. For the protection of the public absolutes such as this are necessary and form an essential part of

Table 2.2 Competency tools for practice and frameworks for education.

Becker (2000)

Core categories

1. Communication skills

2. Psychosocial skills

3. Team skills

4. Physical care skills

5. Life closure skills

6. Intrapersonal skills

De Vleiger et *al.* (2004)

Core categories

Patient:

  1. Nursing observation – comfort measures

  2. Symptom management

  3. Pain management

  4. The terminal phase and death

Family:

  1. Communication issues

  2. The impact of serious illness

  3. Bereavement

General:

  Teamwork

  Self-awareness – ethical issues

good ethical and professional standards (NMC, 2008), yet the objectivity of such judgements is as much open to question as any other system.

At post-registration level the assessment of clinical skills is more complex and is predominantly based around self-judgement validated by educators and only occasionally by practitioners. This assessment usually takes the form of:

■ Reflective essays, diaries and journals – linked to competencies
■ Portfolio development sometimes incorporating competencies
■ Critical incident analysis

This kind of reflective process-centred assessment is indeed one way out of a difficult dilemma, and is popular with HEIs as it makes it much easier and acceptable to validate and assess the work produced against clearly defined academic criteria. It is suggested, however, that the ability to think and write effectively at a given academic standard about clinical issues does not necessarily translate into competence in clinical skills, no matter how articulate, insightful and academically sound the material produced. Higher education remains to this day unsure about validating modes of assessment that put the judgement of competency in the hands of practitioners in a work environment. Currently no form of clinical assessment involving competencies can be said to be wholly objective. Indeed, this may never be fully achievable because of the holistic nature of care delivery and the multiple extraneous variables that can influence such assessment at any one time. Evidence does suggest that an assessor's influence on how a nurse learns when caring for patients and families at the end of life is heavily restricted by such factors (Degner *et al.*, 1991). Perhaps, therefore, universities have a valid point.

Competency in palliative nursing

It is self-evident that many of the cited areas in Tables 2.1 and 2.2 overlap and contribute to the collective expertise and wisdom of a competent practitioner using the palliative approach, but what is there in these tools and frameworks that stands out as essential to palliative nursing? To illustrate this I will take the framework developed from my own research into devising a self assessment competency tool for palliative nursing skills (Becker, 2000). Whilst not definitive, it has nevertheless been extensively evaluated for its efficacy, peer reviewed, published and developed over several years.

Communication skills

A highly developed range of sensitive and facilitative communication skills is to be expected, but is not unique to a palliative setting. Many nurses develop the skills to develop a good rapport with the patient and family, to give important information when requested, and to listen to concerns expressed in a non-judgemental, supportive manner. What makes palliative nursing skills stand out is the further ability to field and respond to sometimes, profound, or rhetorical questions about life and death; to know when to say nothing, because that is the most appropriate response at the time; to use therapeutic comforting touch with confidence; to challenge colleagues who may wish to deny the patient information and perhaps to discuss the imminent death of a loved one with the family. It is this combination of communication skills that makes palliative nursing what it is.

Psychosocial skills

An ability to work with the family, anticipating their needs, putting them in touch with services that can help them and supporting them when appropriate is also important, but not unique to palliative nursing. The psychosocial element of care is often that part which gets delegated to the social worker, who may well have better knowledge of and access to the diversity of support that is available, but like so many members of the healthcare team is transient in nature. It is the nurse who will be there at the most difficult moments helping the patient plan their future care, offering strategies, giving ongoing psychological support and coordinating the other members of the team for the benefit of the patient. It is the trust and confidence built through the ongoing relationship that we have with our patients and the therapeutic use of 'self' that is at the core of the psychosocial approach in palliative nursing.

Teamwork skills

Working closely with other members of the multidisciplinary team is a vital part of good practice inherent within many areas of nursing. The palliative care team, however, is not today confined merely to a charitable hospice environment. It can be found in both acute and community settings and in public and private care. The growth of the nursing role within these teams has been dramatic and continues to represent a much admired model of working (Cox and James, 2004).

Physical care skills

This area is about the knowledge and skills necessary for the delivery of active, hands-on care in whatever setting throughout a wide time span of illness. It is not confined to the last few days of life, but is more focused during this period. In a palliative care context such care embraces a range of skills which are discussed in more detail in Chapter 16, but is centred on the nature of both acute and chronic pain (see Chapter 8). Accurate and holistically oriented pain assessment using a range of tools is essential, as is the ability to utilise these tools in situations where the patient may not be able to respond to questioning (see Chapter 9). It is therefore about the observational skills of the nurse and the intuitive ability to recognise the signs with patients who consistently under-report their pain (Farrer, 2007). It is also about much more than advising our medical colleagues about the appropriate prescription and dosage to manage pain; it also involves the advocacy role that nurses have towards their patients at a time of extreme vulnerability. It is these things that make palliative nursing skills in this area so important to patient care.

Life closure skills

This area is concerned with nursing behaviours and skills which are crucial to the dignity of the patient and family as they perceive it when life is close to an end, and thereafter. Caring for the patient's body and immediate surroundings is probably the most common area of activity in any nurse's daily life. It is also the area that is most taken for granted in all healthcare practice, and the preservation of dignity has become central to government policy for the older person (DoH, 2006).

This area of care has often been referred to as 'basic' care, the implication of which is that it involves unskilled tasks of low importance. Nothing could be further from the truth, and the essential comfort measures that embody such care are of vital importance to the overall wellbeing of our patients and those around the bedside (see Chapter 14). Such care has been described as sacred work, in which the carer enters into the intimate space of the patient and touches parts of the body that are usually private (Wolf, 1989). This is a highly privileged position that demands respect and the high degree of skill and sensitivity to individual need that is so essential when caring for the dying patient.

Intrapersonal skills

One area that is a common thread throughout the cited literature and is seen as a key component in the repertoire of skills needed for successful practice in palliative care is the personal and professional maturity to address the challenging intrapersonal issues intrinsic in caring for dying people and their families.

The need for a nurse to recognise and attempt to understand personal reactions and feelings that are brought forward on occasions is a natural consequence of working with the dying and bereaved and the nurse must be able to reflect on how this affects the care given in sensitive situations. Without doubt this is perhaps the most challenging of all competency areas and plays a significant part in the professional growth of those who choose to work in this field.

The dilemma for nurses is that in order to be truly successful at using the palliative approach there is a need to nurture a level of human contact and relationship that goes beyond the norm, and as such can potentially make the nurse feel very vulnerable emotionally. Such reflective maturity is the domain of experience and learning, but is most certainly not confined to the realms of speciality and is within reach of all nurses.

Assessing your competency in palliative nursing

If you would like to explore your own competency at palliative nursing and to self-assess your skills, then log on to http://www.cancernursing.org/ and register with the website – this will cost you nothing and simply entails giving yourself a username and password to enable you to access the wide range of free courses that are available on this charitable website. Once you have done this you will have access to the 'Introduction to Palliative Care Nursing' course, which has within it the full competency assessment tool mentioned in this chapter (Becker, 2000).

There are a number of ways in which this tool can be used. Firstly take time out and study the statements offered in the tool and score yourself using the grading criteria offered. You may find that you are surprised at how positive your scores are, which is not unusual. It's important to acknowledge this, as nurses often underestimate their perceived level of skills. It is self-affirming and confidence-giving to recognise this. You will probably also score quite low on a number of competency statements. This may be solely due to a lack of exposure to such situations, or perhaps you lack in confidence and knowledge in these areas. These are the ones to highlight for your future development.

Experience has shown that where nurses can complete a self-learning contract and set realistic goals (there is a template offered in the course material) considerable success can be achieved. It is useful to re-score yourself on the assessment tool after completing your objectives. Better still, ask a trusted colleague to also score your competence in practice and discuss this with them. Invariably many nurses often score themselves much lower than a colleague would, and it is useful and affirming to get a comparison.

The success of this approach lies very much in your ability to be both honest and reflective in your assessment. It is undoubtedly challenging, both intellectually and personally, to put one's perceived skills so closely under scrutiny, but if we are to improve the care of the dying in whatever setting it takes place then it is important to define clearly what it is we expect nurses to be able to do and at what standard, and to empower them to be able to move practice forward.

Activities such as this can be cited within professional portfolios as clear evidence of development, can be used within annual appraisal interviews to argue for resources and time to improve skills, can help in the development of job descriptions and will ultimately improve patient care.

Conclusion

Readers may well be wondering why there has been no direct reference to the UK Government's End of Life Care Strategy (DoH, 2008) peppered through-out this chapter. There is no doubting the significant impact that this major initiative is beginning to have on end of life care for all people across the UK, and nurses are playing a key role in its ongoing implementation. It is, however, centred on the overall management and coordination of such care by a range of disciplines in multiple environments and is not specific to nursing *per se*. The Gold Standards Framework (Thomas, 2003) and the Liverpool Care Pathway (Ellershaw and Wilkinson, 2003), which have implicit within them a host of nursing duties are medically led initiatives which concern the whole multidis-ciplinary team. The Preferred Priorities of Care (Storey *et al.*, 2003), which is the only nurse-led initiative, is also designed primarily as a care management tool be used with the patient to help plan and meet their wishes some months prior to their death.

This chapter has, I hope, established that the full range of knowledge, skills and behaviours required for nurses to demonstrate the palliative approach is much broader and deeper than at first realised. Competency attained and used regularly in caring for the dying will carry through a nurse's whole career, simply because people die of many causes in many environments. To have the opportunity to be at the bedside of someone throughout the final months, weeks and moments of their life is indeed a privilege and honour for any carer. For nurses it is both the underpinning and overarching ethos of our profes-sion.

Reflective activity

Read this series of mini case studies carefully and using the competency categories offered indicate the range of skills you feel were used by the nurses within these scenarios.

1. Communication skills
2. Psychosocial skills
3. Team skills

4. Physical care skills
5. Life closure skills
6. Intrapersonal skills

- 'What about my children, what do I tell my girls?' As the tears rolled down her cheek, I passed her a tissue and said 'What do you want to tell them?'. 'I don't know, what do you think?' I paused and gently said 'I think you need to consider yourself first, you've had a lot to take in'. 'Maybe you're right' she said.
- Her breast cancer had spread to her skin, with weeping wounds over her chest, arms, neck and back. She looked at me as I dressed those wounds and said 'You are going to heal them aren't you?'. My heart sank. I smiled, stayed silent and just touched her hand. She knew.
- Anne's eyes are sad, questioning. 'I am just so uncomfortable, this swelling's getting worse. How long will it be before they find out what's wrong with me? I feel helpless. I know what the team suspect, but I feel frustrated that Anne remains in limbo. This once happy and confident woman is just fading away and the doctors remain tight-lipped.
- A mobile lady in her late 30s arrived on the ward. She was terminally ill with widespread cancer and had two young children. After one day she was semi-conscious and hours later totally unresponsive. We were just shocked by it all as she was so young and things had moved so fast. She passed away later that evening and the whole team felt bereft.
- I have a tumour in my spine. Haven't been out of bed for four weeks and the physios insist on using a hoist. Why, for god's sake? I can use my legs now. I am desperate to get home and my wife will never manage a hoist. Then this nurse with a sliding board and a determined smile arrives and takes over. The others don't like it, but three attempts and 40 minutes later and I'm sat in a chair. No contraptions, just a shiny board. Now I can go home. I could have hugged and kissed her.

References

Becker, R. (1999) Teaching communication skills across cultural boundaries. *British Journal of Nursing*, **8**(14), 938–42.

Becker, R. (2000) Competency assessment in palliative nursing . *European Journal of Palliative Care*, **7**(3), 88–91.

Benner, P. (1984) *From Novice to Expert: Excellence and Power in clinical Practice*. Addison-Wesley, California.

Bloom, B. S. (1956) *Taxonomy of Educational Objectives*. Allyn & Bacon, Boston, MA.

Carper, B. (1978) Fundamental patterns of knowing in nursing. *Advances in Nursing Science*, **1**(v),13–23.

Cox, K. and James, V. (2004) Professional boundaries in palliative care. In: *Palliative Care Nursing: Principles and Evidence for Practice* (eds. S. Payne, J. Seymour and C. Ingleton). Open University Press, Milton Keynes.

Davies, B. and Oberle, K. (1990) Dimensions of the supportive role of the nurse in palliative care. *Oncology Nursing Forum*, **17**(1), 87–94.

De Vleiger, M., Gorchs, N., Larkin, P. J. and Porchet, F. (2004) A guide to the development of palliative nurse education in Europe. *Palliative Nurse Education: Report of the EAPC Task Force*. European Association of Palliative Care, Milan.

Degner, L. F., Gow, C. M. and Thompson, L. A. (1991) Critical nursing behaviours in care for the dying. *Cancer Nursing*, **14**(5), 246–53.

Department of Health (2006) Dignity in care Campaign. http://www.dh.gov.uk/en/SocialCare/Socialcarereform/Dignityincare/index.htm. Accessed: 18 February 2009.

Department of Health (2008) *End of Life Care Strategy. Promoting High Quality Care for All Adults at the End of Life*. DoH, London.

Ellershaw, J. and Wilkinson, S. (2003*) Care of the Dying. A Pathway to Excellence*. Oxford University Press, Oxford.

Farrer, K. (2007) Pain control. In: *Palliative Nursing: Improving End of Life Care* (eds. S. Kinghorn and S. Gaines), 2nd edn. Baillière Tindall, Edinburgh.

Heslin, K. and Bramwell, L. (1989) The supportive role of the staff nurse in the hospital palliative care situation. *Journal of Palliative Care*, **5**(3), 20–6.

Nursing and Midwifery Council (2008) *Standards of Conduct, Performance and Ethics for Nurses and Midwives*. NMC, London.

Royal College of Nursing (2002) *A Framework for Nurses Working in Specialist Palliative Care: Competencies Project*. RCN Publications, London.

Royal College of Nursing (2003) *Core Competency Framework for Cancer Nursing: Delivering Effective Patient Care*. RCN Publications, London.

Schon, D. (1987) *Educating the Reflective Practitioner*. Jossey Bass, San Francisco.

Storey, L., Pemberton, C., Howard, A. and O'Donnell, L. (2003) Place of death: Hobson's choice or patient choice? *Cancer Nursing Practice*, **2**(4), 33–8.

Taylor, B., Glass, N., McFarlane, J. and Stirling, C. (1997) Palliative nurses' perceptions of the nature and effects of their work. *International Journal of Palliative Nursing*, **3**(5), 253–8.

Thomas, K. (2003) *Caring for the Dying at Home; Companions on the Journey*. Radcliffe Medical Press, Oxford.

Wolf, Z. R. (1989) Uncovering the hidden work of nursing. *Nursing Health Care*, **10**(8), 462–7.

Original material for this chapter was taken and adapted from the following reference with full permission of the EMAP publishing group:

Becker, R. (2009) Palliative care 2: Exploring the skills that nurses need to deliver high quality care. *Nursing Times*, **105**(14), 18–20.

🖳 Useful websites

Royal College of Nursing: go to specialist palliative care competencies project download: http://www.rcn.org.uk/members/publications/

Department of Health (2009) *Common Core Competences and Principles for Health and Social Care Workers Working with Adults at the End of Life. To Support the National End of Life Care Strategy.* Department of Health, London. Available at: http://www.endoflifecare.nhs.uk/eolc/files/NHS-EoLC_Core_competences-Guide-Jul2009.pdf

DoH EOL Strategy: Department of Health, Dignity in care Campaign. http://www.dh.gov.uk/en/SocialCare/Socialcarereform/Dignityincare/index.htm

📋 Chapter links to the Nursing and Midwifery Council Standards of Conduct, Performance and Ethics for Nurses and Midwives (2008)

Section 1: Make the care of people your first concern, treating them as individuals and respecting their dignity

Treat people as individuals
- You must act as an advocate for those in your care, helping them to access relevant health and social care, information and support

Section 2: Work with others to protect and promote the health and wellbeing of those in your care, their families and carers, and the wider community

Share information with your colleagues
- You must keep your colleagues informed when you are sharing the care of others
- You must facilitate students and others to develop their competence

Work effectively as part of a team
- You must work cooperatively within teams and respect the skills, expertise and contributions of your colleagues

Section 3: Provide a high standard of practice and care at all times

Use the best available evidence
- You must deliver care based on the best available evidence or best practice.

Keep your skills and knowledge up to date
- You must have the knowledge and skills for safe and effective practice when working without direct supervision
- You must recognise and work within the limits of your competence
- You must keep your knowledge and skills up to date throughout your working life
- You must take part in appropriate learning and practice activities that maintain and develop your competence and performance

☑ Self-assessment test

1. Some of the core skills for palliative nursing include:
   A   Pharmacology, diagnostic assessment and treatment
   B   Family care and medical interventions
   C   Counselling and referral skills
   D   Relationship building, physical bedside care and teamwork

2. Competency can best be described as:
   A   Doing a job well
   B   Using experience to perform better
   C   A combination of knowledge, skills and appropriate behaviours
   D   Developing the right attitude for the job

3. Which of these statements best reflects the development of competencies today?
   A   Competencies are essential for everyone because they set a baseline standard
   B   Competency assessment is accurate and reliable in clinical practice
   C   A combination of self- and peer assessment can improve reliability
   D   Reflective essays and portfolios are better ways of determining competence

4. 'A fundamental part of competency assessment is to give managers a tool to discipline someone if they are not doing their job properly.' This statement is:
   A   True
   B   False

5. Which of the following can enhance the development of skills and competency in palliative nursing?
   A A trustworthy mentor
   B Using a simple graduated scale to indicate improvement
   C Competency statements that are clear and unambiguous
   D All of the above

CHAPTER 3

Care pathways

There was a sense of stillness as I walked into the bedroom. She was lying there peaceful, her hair lovingly combed. I looked at her with admiration; she was so brave and had been in control of her illness with her belief in complementary therapies. A small noise distracted me, and I turned my eyes to the right side of the bed, where three of her children were lying on the bed with her and the fourth sat in a chair at her side, holding her hand. I smiled; this was just what she said she wanted. I left the house that day feeling comforted. She had achieved the death she wanted in the place of her choosing and with those she loved all around her.

Learning outcomes

After reading this chapter and completing the reflective activities the learner will be able to:

- Understand the concept of advance care planning and its relevance to achieving quality of life in a palliative context
- Recognise the three main initiatives that comprise the End of Life Care Strategy 2008
- Describe their application in clinical practice

Introduction

The poignant family scene depicted in this beautiful and evocative story gives the reader a sense of sadness and joy in equal measure. Sadness that a much admired and loved woman should die leaving four young children behind, yet joy that she was in the comfort and safety of her own home surrounded by the people she loved and in control of her destiny. From a professional perspective the manner and place of her death is a good illustration of what recent government policy is trying to achieve. One of the key anticipated outcomes of the current End of Life Care Programme (DoH, 2008) is to achieve greater choice for patients in their place of care and place of death. Four years prior to this strategy NICE's *Supportive and Palliative Care Guidance for Adults with Cancer* (2004) emphasised similar:

> A good death is important for patients and families if this can be achieved with dignity, within place of choice and with symptoms well managed.

What are care pathways?

When an anxious patient with a life-threatening illness and their carers ask about diagnosis and prognosis there are often other unspoken questions on their mind beyond 'When will I die?'. Those questions are usually concerned with 'What will happen?'. One way of answering such questions can be by talking about patterns of illness and common symptoms suffered to give an indicator of what may happen. These trajectories are generic in nature and can only provide an indicator to the patient, but they do allow for common patterns to be recognised and planned for by health professionals. Such patterns can help clinicians plan and deliver appropriate care that integrates active palliative management of their illness in many different settings. If patients and their carers can gain a better understanding by considering illness trajectories this can help them feel in greater control of their situation and empower them to cope with its demands.

It is this simple thesis that is behind the development of care pathways for end of life care in the UK today and which has the potential to radically improve care for the dying in multiple environments. Quite simply, far too many people still die an undignified death with uncontrolled symptoms, in settings that are not conducive to their needs and with staff who either fail to understand those needs or who are unable to fulfil them due to other service priorities. It is the hospice movement which has given us the expertise in this area over the last 50 years and the best practice lessons and evidence base that has been developed is now being transferred into other settings for the benefit of these disadvantaged dying.

Patient choice

The ever-increasing focus on patient choice and self-determination within health and social care settings has added to the impetus for standardising care plans. Indeed, there is pressure worldwide to achieve this in palliative care (Saunders, 2004). In the UK there have been many initiatives to promote choice over place of death (Commission for Health Improvement/Audit Commission, 2001; DoH, 2000, 2003; National Institute for Clinical Excellence, 2004; National Council for Palliative Care, 2005). Within these initiatives, generalists as well as specialists are expected to acquire the necessary skills to facilitate this choice.

What has emerged from these policy developments is the End of Life Care programme, which was set up in England in 2005 to promote three initiatives which had been independently developed to facilitate good practice for dying patients: the Gold Standards Framework (Thomas, 2003), Liverpool Care Pathway (Ellershaw and Wilkinson, 2003) and the Preferred Priorities of Care Document (Storey *et al.*, 2003). The Preferred Priorities of Care (PPC) document, a type of advanced care plan (Seymour and Henry, 2007) was developed as a tool to record patient and carer choice. It allows reviews at different points in the pathway of care, records services available and services being accessed, and reasons for changes. This document is patient held, and is intended to be used in a variety of differing health and social care settings. It therefore provides empowerment for patients in communicating their wishes wherever they go.

The Liverpool Care Pathway

The specialist palliative care team at the Royal Liverpool University Hospitals and the Team at the Marie Curie Centre Liverpool established the LCP Project as a means by which the expertise in terminal care developed by hospices could be transferred into mainstream healthcare environments, where most people die. It is a multi-professional document which provides an evidence-based framework for care during the last few weeks or days of someone's life and guidance on the different aspects of care required, including comfort measures, anticipatory prescribing of medicines and discontinuation of inappropriate interventions. Additionally, psychological and spiritual care and family support are included.

The holistic emphasis supports the palliative care philosophy entirely and emphasises to the care team that dying is more than the effects of a disease process and is a normal life event which affects the whole person (WHO, 2002). For it to be successful the team first has to acknowledge that the patient is dying. This may sound obvious, but the diagnosis of dying is a subject that is avoided by many medical practitioners because of its contradiction to their stated aims of preserving life. Recognising futility is at the core of such decision making and it is good education that gives the confidence for this to happen. Nurses are only slightly better equipped than our medical colleagues to assist with such decisions by virtue of the holistic caring philosophy that underpins all nursing practice and acknowledges dying as part of this, but there is a real need for better preparation.

The documentation is designed to be used by the whole care team and replaces all previous case notes, thereby avoiding the often used criticism of many such initiatives that the bureaucracy is overburdening in busy environments. An audit of existing practice takes place prior to the implementation of the care pathway to provide a baseline for future measurement of the outcomes and an education strategy for the team is integral to its structure.

What it is/should be

- Capable of reflecting a range of patient needs in a palliative context
- Reflects an expected course of events towards the end of life
- A means of proactively managing end of life care
- A means to demonstrate high-quality consistent care of the dying
- A way of identifying the individual needs of the dying patient
- A means of demonstrating and achieving integrated team work
- For patients of all diagnoses and not just cancer

What is isn't

- The perfect tool
- An exercise in 'tick box' care management
- A straitjacket restricting practice
- Something you must do
- Something one person alone can do
- It is not about reducing nursing care
- It is definitely not 'speeding up' the dying phase

There are three sections to the pathway:

1. Initial assessment and care
2. Ongoing assessment and care
3. Care after death

Each section has it own colour-coded documents to identify which discipline has completed it and has a list of questions to be asked to ascertain the patient's needs. One of the words that crops up in the documentation frequently is 'variance', which is an audit-related term that means the recording of changes in the patient's condition which have an impact on the care delivered. For example – if pain is no longer controlled or a catheter is no longer draining this is a deviation from what you have been recording and is known as a variance. This variance should be recorded within the documentation and acted upon accordingly.

Essentially this is no different from using the nursing process, which has a systematic approach to the assessment, planning, implementation and evaluation of care in a cycle which is continually being reviewed and updated. What causes confusion is the choice of words and what some see as the imposition of more new and unfamiliar documentation. In reality, there should be less bureaucracy and not more, because all other case notes are taken away when the decision is made to put someone on the pathway. One further cause of concern is what should happen if the patient should recover and be able to receive fluids. Quite simply, the patient should be removed from the pathway until is agreed once more that they are within a terminal care state. As Chapter 5 on ethics states clearly, no patient who is thirsty and capable of drinking should ever be denied fluids simply because a care management tool says otherwise.

The Gold Standards Framework

The impetus behind the creation of this care management tool was the desire to support those who choose to die at home by equipping the primary care teams with the knowledge, skills and means by which they can plan effective care in advance of the terminal phase according to the patients' wishes. It is the brainchild of Dr Keri Thomas, a GP, and is now being rolled out across the UK to over 2000 GP practices (Thomas, 2005).

The GSF is an evidence-based programme of assessment and care which provides a home pack for patients to facilitate the sharing of information between health professionals. The aim is to improve and optimise quality of life for the dying and those important to them in the last 6–12 months of life. Each GP practice that elects to take on the scheme is required to nominate a key nurse and doctor for each patient who is placed on a locally held register. From then on, monthly team meetings are held to review the patient's situation and to monitor their illness trajectory. Every six months a larger meeting takes place to enable the sharing of experiences from the team and for protocols to be modified or stepped up. This is where the range of assessments that have been carried out (which can include pain, diet, mobility, and other symptoms) are scrutinised and evaluated. The 'toolkit', as it is called, covers seven key areas:

- Communication
- Control of symptoms
- Continuity of care
- Coordination
- Care support
- Care of the dying
- Continued learning

The education and support network that goes with this initiative is within the NHS and offers help to strategic health authorities, primary care trusts and cancer networks. The focus is very much on forward planning and good team-work to enable a death at home with good support, avoiding the need for last-minute hospital admissions. Government support is strong and GSF is seen as a key part of the End of Life Care Strategy. The downside is that there is no compulsion for GP practices to adopt GSF, despite its proven benefits. The uptake of it has been enthusiastic in some areas, with almost saturation cover-age, whilst some neighbouring trusts have ignored it altogether. For patients, access to the programme very much depends on where they live – a situa-tion which once more creates the phenomenon known as a 'postcode lottery', which is just what it was hoped would be avoided.

Preferred Priorities in Care

The figures published for those who would chose to die at home if they could (56%) and those who currently achieve this goal (20%) (NCPC, 2005) make for shameful reading in a country that has led the way internationally in the provision of specialist services in palliative care. We may have some of the best palliative care academics, clinicians and educators in the world here in the UK, and the most integrated services, but we still have a long way to go to influence mainstream practice in where and how people die. The ideal of choice remains just an ideal for many people. Empowerment is perhaps one of the most effective means of promoting choice, and this is the rationale behind the development of the PPC documentation. The idea came to fruition within the Lancashire and Cumbria Cancer Network, and its primary spokesperson, developer and champion is Les Storey, an experienced nurse, academic and educator.

The aim is to put the patient at the centre of any plan of care, with the intention of promoting control and autonomy for them, from the early stages of the pallia-tive experience right through to death and thereafter, in the place of their choosing. The documentation is held by the patient and follows them through their illness wherever they go, with a transparency in choice and preferences for all health professionals (Storey *et al.*, 2003). There are four parts to the plan:

- **Section 1**: Family profile – this gives details of the person's dependence and identifies who the key carers are.
- **Section 2**: Details of the person's preferences are recorded here, along with the discussions that led to the choices made. This can include where they wish to die, who they would like with them, what interventions they would like and what they would not like, and who their advocates (who hold the documents) are.
- **Section 3**: Details of health assessments such as pain, diet, mobility, and other symptoms, are included here and are available for whatever service is delivering the care.
- **Section 4**: This final section allows for the recording of changes in care by health professionals as time moves on.

It is made very clear to patients that although the document is a clear expression of wishes it may not be possible to honour all the elements recorded due to factors such as a rapid change in condition, a change in carer circumstances or limited resources. As a statement of intent, however, it is invaluable, as it facilitates open and honest discussion between all concerned and can help families know exactly what someone would want if and when they lose capacity.

 Reflective activity

Which of these three projects is operative in your area? When you find this information ask about the main benefits it has brought and what the difficulties have been in implementing the projects. Make notes on this and see if there are any common denominators.

Education in support of end of life care

Whilst all three of these initiatives have programmes of education for health professionals integral to their implementation, there is little if any such education at pre-registration level. Medical education has had the palliative approach integrated into the training of all doctors in the UK since 1992 (Palliative Medicine Curriculum, 1992). Since that time the average number of hours devoted to such education has increased significantly (Field and Bee Wee, 2002). By contrast, however, the formal teaching of the palliative approach in UK nursing faculties remains *ad hoc* at best (Lloyd Williams and Field, 2002) and no such national imperative yet exists (Cooley, 2004), despite government recognition of the need (DoH, 2004). This a shameful state of affairs and unless the Nursing and Midwifery Council takes this issue forward with clear, unequivocal mandatory recommendations it will never significantly improve. The statutory curricular requirements over three years' training to produce safe and effective nurses are immense, and universities struggle to meet them as they are. It is no surprise therefore that those elements of care such as palliation, whilst acknowledged as important, are subsumed within modular schemes with only the occasional learning outcome appearing within a raft of other deserving priorities.

Conclusion

The long-term efficacy of these initiatives is yet to be seen, but if used with care and compassion as intended, with an emphasis on individualised care, they have the potential to transform care of the dying in multiple environments. It has to be remembered that they are only tools and not a universal panacea or an outcome in themselves. Success very much relies on the education of the professionals who use them and their perception of the tool as something of use and not a hindrance. The idea of measurable outcomes in end of life care is a seductive one that has captured the minds of many academics and clinicians in recent years. From a purely economic perspective it can be argued that unless sound quantitative as well as qualitative evidence is gathered to demonstrate the worth of palliative interventions then future funding from cash-strapped governments might be increasingly hard to get and the advances achieved in how we now use the palliative approach will be lost in the complex politics of healthcare. In other words, the money will go elsewhere.

It can also be argued that to perceive end of life care in such a way is reductionist and dangerous, in that the only truly valid measure of success is that the patient has a good death as defined by them. Whilst certain common denominators can be tracked and used for care planning, the subjective, emotive, psychosocial and existential elements will always defy analysis by accountants and it is these elements that make up a large part of such care and are of primary concern to nurses. Notably it is the two medically led tools – the LCP and GSF – which have received the highest profile and funding. The PPC, on the other hand, which is nurse-led with patient-held documentation through all stages of dying, has received little support across the UK despite its clear benefits to give choice and empowerment directly to the patient; something which is central to the End of Life Care Strategy.

Nurses have a vital role in the shaping of services for the dying over the next decade and beyond. Much of the success of government involvement in care of the dying will be down to nurses and not our medical colleagues, despite their stronger position as clinical leads. It is nurses who will review, document, evaluate and deliver the hands-on care on a day-to-day basis and it is nurses who will work closest with the family and be in the most informed position to determine for the team whether the 'good death' in the place of choosing was achieved or not. Care pathways have an important role to play in this and it is nursing's duty to ensure that the humanity of care is valued when the outcomes of these initiatives are evaluated.

References

Cooley, C. (2004) Core skills nursing cancer. *International Cancer Nursing News*, **16**(2), 45.

Commission for Health Improvement/Audit Commission (2001) *National Service Framework Assessments No.1:NHS cancer care in England and Wales*. CHI/AC, London.

Department of Health (2000) *The NHS Cancer Plan: a plan for Investment, a Plan for Reform*. DoH, London.

Department of Health (2003) *Building on the Best: Choice, Responsiveness and Equity in the NHS*. DoH, London.

Department of Health (2004) *Supportive and Palliative Care Guidance for Adults with Cancer*. NICE, London.

Department of Health (2008) *End of Life Care Strategy. Promoting High Quality Care for All Adults at the End of Life*. DoH, London.

Ellershaw, J. and Wilkinson, S. (2003) *Care of the Dying. A Pathway to Excellence*. Oxford University Press, Oxford.

Field, D. and Bee Wee (2002) Preparation for palliative care: teaching about death, dying and bereavement in UK medical schools 2000-2001. *Medical Education*, **36**, 561–7.

Lloyd Williams, M. and Field, D. (2002) Are undergraduate nurses taught palliative care during their training? *Nurse Education Today*, 22 Oct (7), 589–92.

National Council for Palliative Care (2005) *Priorities and Preference for End of Life Care*. Occasional Paper NCPC, London.

National Institute for Clinical Excellence (2004) *Improving Supportive and Palliative Care for Adults with Cancer: The Manual*. NICE, London.

Palliative Medicine Curriculum for Medical Students, General Professional Training and Specialist Training (1992) Association for Palliative Medicine. Cited in National Council for Hospice and Specialist Palliative Care Services (1996) *Education in Palliative Care*. Occasional Paper 9.

Saunders, C. (2004) Preface. In: *Palliative Care. The Solid Facts* (eds. E. Davies and J. Higginson). World Health Organization, Geneva.

Storey, L., Pemberton, C., Howard, A. and O'Donnell, L. (2003) Place of death: Hobson's choice or patient choice? *Cancer Nursing Practice*, **2**(4), 33–8.

Seymour, J. and Henry, C. (2007) *Advanced Care Planning: A Guide for Health and Social Care Staff*. NHS End of Life Care Programme.

Thomas, K. (2003) *Caring for the Dying at Home; Companions on the Journey*. Radcliffe Medical Press, Oxford.

Thomas, K. (2005) *Background to GSF*. http://www.goldstandardsframework.nhs.uk/. Accessed: 1 October 2009.

World Health Organization (2002) *National Cancer Control Programmes: Policies and Managerial Guidelines*, 2nd edn. WHO, Geneva.

World Health Organization (2009) http://www.who.int/cancer/palliative/definition/en/. Accessed: 30 September 2009.

Useful websites

Department of Health End of Life Strategy; Department of Health Dignity in Care Campaign. http://www.dh.gov.uk/en/SocialCare/Socialcarereform/Dignityincare/index.htm

End of Life Care Strategy
http://www.endoflifecareforadults.nhs.uk/eolc/

Essence of Care
http://www.dh.gov.uk/en/Publicationsandstatistics/Publications/PublicationsPolicyAndGuidance/DH_4005475

Gold Standards Framework
http://www.goldstandardsframework.nhs.uk/

Liverpool Care Pathway
http://www.liv.ac.uk/mcpcil/liverpool-care-pathway/documentation-lcp.htm

Preferred Priorities of Care
http://www.cancerlancashire.org.uk/ppc.html

Chapter links to the Nursing and Midwifery Council Standards of Conduct, Performance and Ethics for Nurses and Midwives (2008)

Section 1: Make the care of people your first concern, treating them as individuals and respecting their dignity

Collaborate with those in your care
■ You must listen to the people in your care and respond to their concerns and preferences

- You must support people in caring for themselves to improve and maintain their health
- You must recognise and respect the contribution that people make to their own care and wellbeing
- You must make arrangements to meet people's language and communication needs
- You must share with people, in a way they can understand, the information they want or need to know about their health

Work effectively as part of a team

- You must work cooperatively within teams and respect the skills, expertise and contributions of your colleagues
- You must consult and take advice from colleagues when appropriate
- You must make a referral to another practitioner when it is in the best interests of someone in your care

Section 3: Provide a high standard of practice and care at all times

Use the best available evidence

- You must deliver care based on the best available evidence or best practice
- You must ensure any advice you give is evidence-based if you are suggesting healthcare products or services
- You must ensure that the use of complementary or alternative therapies is safe and in the best interests of those in your care

☑ Self-assessment test

1. An end of life care pathway is:
    A A checklist of 'do's and 'don't's for the healthcare team
    B A statement of preference in care
    C A common core of symptoms and issues that enable a plan of care
    D A tool for advance care planning that respects choice and autonomy

2. Which of these statements is not true?
    A Advance care plans give greater autonomy for patients
    B Medical priorities take precedence over care pathway tools
    C Used wisely such plans have the potential to help many people die a better death
    D When someone is on the pathway they are on it until death

3. The End of Life Care Strategy is:
   A   A government project to evaluate care management tools
   B   A means by which the three project leads can advance their careers
   C   A coordinated national initiative to improve choice in place of dying, dignity and support
   D   A valiant but disjointed attempt at taking the hospice model and applying it elsewhere

4. The reported percentage who say they wish to die at home in the UK is:
   A   56%
   B   65%
   C   46%
   D   73%

5. Some of the criticisms of care pathways include:
   A   They dehumanise care into a mechanistic process
   B   They are cheaper than alternatives because of less bureaucracy
   C   They are an exercise in tick box management
   D   Pathways speed up the dying process

CHAPTER 4

Palliative care for all diagnoses

Bert had renal failure and cardiac failure and now needed a leg amputation for gangrene. His prognosis was poor and he knew it, his wife and son had left him and he had lost his job. All in all he was in complete despair. I took him outside for a cigarette – his last remaining comfort – and tried very hard to give Bert some hope as he faced his surgery. We sat in silence. The door opened and out came a young physiotherapist who walked past carrying a hacksaw. Bert and I caught each others eye and we both dissolved into raucous laughter.

 Learning outcomes

After reading this chapter and completing the reflective activities the learner will be able to:

- Understand the need for better palliative care provision for patients of all diagnoses
- Describe the complex professional issues that have to be addressed in order to provide palliative care for different diagnoses
- Identify the nursing issues at the end of life for the most common conditions where palliative care needs are greatest

Introduction

Bert's awful situation is tragic indeed; his life has fallen apart around him and he is facing his mortality the only way he knows how. His needs are manifest and whilst the imminent surgery may well give him some extra time to live, it is the quality of the life he has left and how he will cope with the issues he has to face that will determine whether he dies with dignity in the manner of his choosing. The nurse looking after him recognises this and their mutual understanding and affinity for this reality is quite clear, which is exactly why in the context of the moment when the physiotherapist walks by with the saw in her hand they both use laughter as a valid and useful coping strategy.

It is not the intention of this chapter to enter into a descriptive dialogue related to the complex aetiology and physiology of each condition, or indeed the active management of the most common conditions. There are a good number of excellent texts already on the market that can fulfil this role. This book will confine itself to a brief exploration of the most common symptomatology that is likely to be encountered close to the end of life and the key nursing issues that arise from these in clinical practice.

The current situation

The evidence base we now have to support care for the dying has grown enormously over the last 50 years and the art and science of palliative care have demonstrated quite clearly that although much of this knowledge has been gained through work with cancer patients, the needs of people like Bert are no different regardless of his diagnosis. It is one of the ultimate ironies of the palliative care movement that its philosophy has never been anything other than inclusive of all dying people, yet it is the development of the modern hospice building and its bias towards cancer patients that has in part led to the perception that those dying of other equally deserving diagnoses are somehow disadvantaged. Whether that is genuinely true is a matter for conjecture, but in the UK there is no denying the fact that it is the charitable status and independence of the majority of the hospice movement from government control that has caused this to happen and is both what keeps hospices alive and thriving and conversely makes them open to the criticism of being elitist and for the cancer sufferer only.

This is a paradox that has been brought sharply into focus in the last five years in particular as for the first time ever government policy has stepped into the specialist palliative care arena and decided that the needs of the many who die in institutions and at home outweigh the needs of the few who die in hospices and something needs to be done to correct this imbalance. The *End of Life Care Strategy* (DoH, 2008) is the culmination of this thinking and it remains to be seen over the next decade whether this noble intent can effectively be translated into the long-term vision of palliative care for all.

What can specialist palliative care offer the generalist?

■ Expertise – dealing with complex physical, psychological, spiritual or social problems in the face of death

- Determining whether death is certain or likely – the diagnosis of dying
- Familiarity in talking about death and dying
- Familiarity in thinking through the difficult ethical issues at end of life
- Skilled symptom control
- Expertise in the care of actively dying patients and their needs

There are a number of reasons why the specialist palliative care movement has been slow to address the non-cancer agenda. Firstly, whereas those dying of cancer follow an illness trajectory that is more or less predictable and time limited, the needs of those with chronic cardiac failure, chronic obstructive airways disease, endocrine disorders and any number of degenerative conditions are open-ended, from several days or weeks through to many years. Essentially they are chronic illnesses and modern medicine can mitigate the worst of the symptomatology to improve life quality up to a point and in doing so prolong life for sometimes large and indeterminate periods. What eventually ends the person's life may therefore be little to do with their original diagnosis, but a consequence of their restricted lifestyle. The fears are that funding and resources will be inadequate to deal with this and inpatient demand for beds in hospices will multiply beyond what can be managed.

The reality of such fears has thankfully not been realised and it is apparent that the existing services for the majority of patients of differing diagnoses have no intention of making such demands, but what is needed is the means by which they can access specialist help and advice when needed to improve care for those dying in whatever environment. As can be seen from the above bullet list, many of the skills are immediately transferable and one of the main challenges that hospices now have to face is how to educate, support and work with the many disparate teams of health and social care professionals who are calling on them for advice and counsel.

How should palliative care respond to high level of need?

Education is the mantra on everyone's lips. Develop education services to match the need and skill the generalists in the principles and practice of using the palliative approach and problem will be solved. Idealistic – yes, simplistic and naïve – most definitely. The UK has the best integrated education services for palliative care professionals anywhere in the world, with a proliferation of postgraduate opportunities and a vast range of non accredited education provided by universities and hospices (Becker, 2004). What's more, it has been this way for the last 30 years. Countless thousands of nurses, doctors and allied health professionals have attended such education and benefited from the knowledge gained. Almost without exception that education has been non-cancer-focused so that the broad principles can be taken and applied to individual circumstances and practice. Has it made a difference to care? That is a more difficult question to answer and evaluative evidence of broad-based competency translating into better outcomes for the patient remains an elusive goal for all educationalists. One thing is certain, however, there are many thousands of families and patients who can anecdotally give testament to the value of the palliative care they have received from experienced and knowledgeable practitioners.

We also know that much more needs to be done, and as long as both hospices in general and universities continue to pay lip service to the development of palliative-related skills and knowledge by refusing to see such education as a core and essential component of service development and not just as a value-added adjunct, then change will be slow indeed. Education is a two-way process and it is just as important for specialist palliative care providers to learn about heart failure, dementia and chronic respiratory disease as it is for these teams in hospitals and the community to learn about the palliative approach.

Other options

Different models of service provision merit further exploration and the idea of one-off consultations between the referring team and the palliative care team has met with some success. Also possible are short-term interventions from the palliative care team, with re-referral if needed. Whatever model is used there needs to be a continuing commitment from specialist palliative care providers because of the complexity of the need.

Criteria for supportive/palliative care

One of the key issues is deciding not only who should get the care but when it should be instigated. The science of diagnosing dying is a subjective one, so criteria need to be agreed to make this happen. The Gold Standards Framework has within it a suggested three-question criterion that is simple to understand and represents a good step forward for clinical practice in many environments (GSF, 2009).

1. The surprise question 'Would you be surprised if this patient were to die in the next 6–12 months?' – an intuitive question integrating co-morbidity, social and other factors. If you would not be surprised, then what measures might be taken to improve their quality of life now and in preparation for the dying stage? The surprise question can be applied to years/months/weeks/days and trigger the appropriate actions. The aim is to enable the right thing to happen at the right time; e.g. if days, then begin a Care Pathway for the Dying. Some clinicians find it easier to ask themselves 'Would you be surprised if this patient were still alive in 6–12 months?'.
2. Choice/need: the patient with advanced disease makes a choice for comfort care only, not 'curative' treatment, or is in special need of supportive/palliative care, e.g. refusing renal transplant.
3. Clinical indicators: general and specific indicators of advanced disease for each of the three main end of life patient groups - cancer, organ failure, elderly frail/ dementia

 Reflective activity

On your current and next clinical placement make a list of the range of conditions you encounter over a period of several weeks and take the three prognostic indicators listed above and ask yourself which patients fit one, two or all three of the criteria. This should give you some idea of palliative care needs in different environments.

Best practice with the most common conditions

End stage heart failure

Two of the key documents that have provided the impetus for addressing palliative care needs in this area are the National Institute for Clinical Excellence guidelines on chronic heart failure which state 'issues of sudden death and living with uncertainty are pertinent to all patients with heart failure. Opportunities to discuss these issues should be available at all stages of care' (NICE, 2005) and the National Service Framework for Chronic Heart Disease (CHD) (NSF, 2000), which recommends a palliative approach in managing end stage heart failure and identifies 'open communication about disease outcomes should be offered to all patients suffering from heart failure'.

The main symptoms include:

- Breathlessness
- Oedema

- Light-headedness, muscle wasting and fatigue
- Nausea and anorexia
- Taste disturbance
- Anxiety and/or depression
- Pain

(McGavigan and Dunn, 2005)

The psychological impact of severe CHD on the individual can be immense, with a real risk of depression about the impact of the physical limitations imposed on their life. They are less able to care for themselves and unable to work or pursue hobbies, their social life suffers and they can be very anxious about what will happen in the future as symptoms begin to worsen.

Nursing issues at the end of life include:

- Correct positioning and the possible use of oxygen, inhalers and nebulisers for dyspnoea
- Assessment of need for treatment of oedema via the local oedema nurse specialist who can advise on a range of options
- Monitoring of urine output due to the prescription of diuretics
- Support when mobilising due to the risk of postural hypotension and monitoring of blood pressure
- High-calorie low-salt diet and food supplements to offset the effects of muscle wasting
- Regular mouth care
- The pacing of mobilising activities built around the patients needs with regular rests
- Monitoring of the efficacy of all prescriptions
- Vomit bowls at the bedside
- Psychological support including good active listening for concerns, support of the family and activities to occupy time
- Alert for enduring signs of possible depression, e.g. consistent low mood, early morning waking, disturbed sleep pattern. Assessment by a psychiatrist may be needed
- Full holistic assessment and management for associated pain (see Chapters 6, 7 and 8)

Chronic Obstructive Pulmonary Disease (COPD)

It is estimated that about 13% of adult disability is the result of respiratory disease in the UK and it is a leading cause of morbidity and mortality, yet it is the most under-funded and poorly recognised of all the chronic diseases that merit a palliative approach (Buckley, 2008).

Elkington's research (Elkington *et al.*, 2005) into the health and social care needs of COPD patients in the last year of life demonstrated that these people:

■ Experience a heavy burden of symptoms in last year of life
■ Feel socially isolated
■ Have limited contact with health services
■ Have rare involvement with specialist respiratory or specialist palliative care nurses
■ Have overall poorly coordinated care

The primary symptomatology associated with COPD is dyspnoea, pain, cough, insomnia and low mood.

Nursing issues at the end of life include:

■ Management of breathlessness by the use of
 – Careful positioning
 – Oxygen therapy
 – Bronchodilator therapy – inhalers and nebulisers
■ Passive exercises
■ Monitoring of urine output due to possible diuresis
■ Supportive psychological care at the bedside, including good active listening for concerns both physical and existential
■ Physiotherapy exercises regarding coughing
■ Full holistic assessment and management for associated pain (see Chapters 6, 7 and 8)

Neurodegenerative disease

There are a wide range of neurodegenerative diseases that can affect both adults and children, and in the main they cause a gradual deterioration of psychomotor function and sometimes cognitive function. The end result of this progressive loss is an increasing dependence on family and eventually healthcare professionals. Whilst we have developed a good level of knowledge in the management of these conditions, little is known as to their causation and this can and does lead to much anxiety and negativity from all carers, as there is no hope of cure offered to sufferers. Equally, the progression of many of these conditions is so variable from person to person that it can be difficult to give a sufferer any indication of their expected level of disability and of course ultimately a prognosis.

Multiple sclerosis is a good case in point. Even diagnosis itself can be difficult, as much symptomatology is so subtle that it is either ignored for long periods by the person, who adjusts their life around the symptoms, or the GP considers (quite rightly) many other differential diagnoses before referral to a neurologist, many months from first presentation. Sufferers of the more aggressive types of MS can go from full mobility to death within months, whereas others receive regular treatment and monitoring and maintain a full active lifestyle for many years.

The most commonly encountered neurodegenerative diseases include:

- Multiple sclerosis (MS)
- Motor neurone disease (MND) – also known as amyotrophic lateral sclerosis (AMS). American texts in particular use this term
- Huntingdon's disease – used to be known as Huntingdon's chorea
- Parkinson's disease
- Cerebro-vascular accidents (CVA) – strokes

The most common symptoms associated with these conditions include:

- Pain – both nociceptive and neuropathic in origin (see Chapter 8 for an explanation of these concepts)
- Respiratory difficulties – breathlessness and dyspnoea
- Dysarthria and anarthria – speech problems due to loss of motor function as a result of disease progression
- Salivary dribbling
- Bladder problems – incontinence and/or intermittent dribbling
- Bowel problems – constipation in particular
- Depression – a long-term risk with the possibility of suicide being considered at some point

Nursing issues at the end of life include:

- Full holistic assessment and management for associated pain (see Chapters 6, 7 and 8)
- Awareness of the need for neuropathic pain to be managed differently to nociceptive pain
- Management of breathlessness and dyspnoea by the use of
  - Careful positioning
  - Oxygen therapy
  - Bronchodilator therapy – inhalers and nebulisers
  - Awareness of the risk of aspiration
- Incontinence – use of a variety of incontinence aids to improve life quality, i.e. pads, specialist underwear and catheterisation as a last resort. Seek the advice of your local incontinence nurse specialist

- Active catheter management including cleansing to reduce the risk of a urinary tract infection, monitoring for leakage or obstruction and possibly irrigation. Antibiotics may be appropriate depending on how close to death the team consider the patient to be
- Bowel management – at the end of life active intervention to clear constipation is inappropriate, intrusive and unnecessary; however, earlier in the illness trajectory attention to diet and the use of laxatives can relieve much potential distress
- Creative attention to communication difficulties – seek the advice of your local speech therapist
- Cognitive difficulties – memory loss and behavioural issues should be anticipated alongside anxiety and frustration. This merits careful use of listening and attending skills combined with supportive teamwork and agreed strategies with the family to preserve dignity and personhood
- Poor nutrition – at the end of life this is generally not an issue, but where the person is capable of eating then high-calorie meals and supplements, well presented, are the key to success
- Dribbling – this can be managed successfully today by the use of sublingual or transdermal hyoscine hydrobromide. Sometimes amitriptyline is successful, but beware of the risk of a dry and uncomfortable mouth
- Mouth care – regular cleansing and attention to lip condition

Dementia

This debilitating condition is characterised by the progressive impairment of both short- and long-term memory, impaired judgement, and an overall loss of most cognitive function. There is little doubt that it is one of the most distressing conditions one can encounter in clinical practice and for the sufferer has been described as a 'living death'. For the family it's an emotional and physical rollercoaster of watching the gradual decline of a loved one into someone who is unrecognisable in terms of their personality, which is all but destroyed. Issues of loss and grief are manifest with family members before the person dies and for the sufferer there can be occasional episodes of insight that render them aware to some degree of their predicament and which cause much distress.

Recent work evaluating the impact of the National Service Framework for older people and its impact on dementia sufferers (NSF, 2009) has resulted in the development of a National Dementia Strategy (NDS, 2009) in an endeavour to promote research and policy for what is one of the biggest healthcare challenges now facing the UK and beyond. Guidelines produced by the National Institute for Health and Clinical Excellence (NICE, 2007) can give us a good indicator of the complex care issues involved.

The most commonly reported symptoms suffered by the person with dementia in the last year of life were confusion (83%), urinary incontinence (72%), pain (64%), low mood (61%), constipation (59%) and loss of appetite (57%) (McCarthy *et al.*, 1997). Furthermore, there may also be issues with nutrition and hydration, decubitus ulcers, swallowing, mobility and aspiration pneumonia (Buckley, 2008).

Nursing issues at the end of life include:

- Full holistic assessment and management for associated pain (see Chapters 6, 7 and 8)
- Awareness of the need to use observational pain assessment scales rather than patient reporting scales. A full review of these can be found at Zwakhalen *et al.* (2006)
- Management of breathlessness and dyspnoea by the use of:
  - Careful positioning
  - Oxygen therapy
  - Bronchodilator therapy – inhalers and nebulisers
  - Awareness of the risk of aspiration
- Incontinence – regular toileting regime (e.g. 3 hourly) helps greatly; however, use of a variety of incontinence aids may improve life quality, e.g. pads, specialist underwear and catheterisation as a last resort. Seek the advice of your local incontinence nurse specialist
- Bowel management – at the end of life active intervention to clear constipation is inappropriate, intrusive and unnecessary; however, earlier in the illness trajectory attention to diet and the use of laxatives can relieve much potential distress
- Poor nutrition – at the end of life this is generally not an issue, but where the person is capable of eating, then high-calorie meals and supplements, well presented, are the key to success. The ethics and practicality of using a nasogastric tube or percutaneous endoscopic gastrostomy for feeding have to be carefully balanced against perceived quality of life
- Decubitus ulcers – these arise as a result of poor pressure area care; therefore the use of a regularly reviewed pressure assessment risk tool such as that devised by Judy Waterlow (2009), which is in common use across the UK, will help to monitor risk

⏳ Reflective point

Many sufferers of dementia are cared for in environments that are not suited to their needs and are significantly disadvantaged, being seen as the 'difficult patient' due to the behavioural problems. The next time you come across this, find out how you can contact the local mental health specialist services who will have experts in this area and ask them to help advise in care management.

Conclusion

We have a long way to go yet before services for non-cancer patients in the last months of life (and their families) have their needs for physical, psychological and social support fully met. This is a difficult issue to resolve, not least because of the simple fact that most of the specialist services for palliative care that can help and advise are in the hands of the charitable sector and not the mainstream NHS. Control, therefore, over service improvement and developments rest with a collaborative approach that draws in this sector with concrete incentives and yet recognises and respects their independence. It is fair to say that funding to support the development of services for the non-cancer patient has not been forthcoming beyond the initial push of the End of Life Care Strategy (DoH, 2008). As long as government is content to leave this to the vagaries of the charitable sector and their uncertain funding in difficult financial times, instead of securing long-term, ring-fenced primary funding, radical improvement will be unlikely to happen.

What has to be decided is the future role of palliative care services in improving the care of these patients. One response has been to develop alternatives to what might be described as 'full palliative care', with the full multidisciplinary team being involved and with an open-ended commitment. As this model from the Royal College of Physicians Report of 2007 suggests (RCP, 2007), some will only need a one-off consultation between, for example, the heart failure nurse and the palliative care nurse, others may need short-term interventions with re-referral when needed, and a minority will need the full package. Many teams work in this way in the cancer sector already.

Addressing the needs of non-cancer patients raises fundamental questions about the purpose and core values of palliative care as it is currently organised and perceived in the UK. There is a definite need for more research into the palliative needs of this large group of dying people and into developing realistic ways of meeting those needs. In the meantime, student nurses and all healthcare professionals will encounter these people on a daily basis and will hopefully deliver care based on need, not diagnosis, so that the aim of giving the person a dignified end to their life in the place of their choice is achieved as closely as possible.

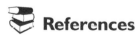 **References**

Addington, H. and Higginson, I. J. (eds.) (2001) *Palliative Care for Non-cancer Patients*. Oxford University Press, Oxford.

Becker, R. (2004) An international perspective in education in cancer and palliative care. In: *Delivering Cancer and Palliative Care Education* (eds. L. Foyle and J. Hostad). Radcliffe Press, Oxford.

Buckley, J. (2008) Palliative issues in common diseases. In: *Palliative Care: an Integrated Approach*. Wiley Blackwell, Chichester.

Department of Health (2008) *End of Life Care Strategy. Promoting High Quality Care for All Adults at the End of Life*. DoH, London.

Elkington, H., White, P., Addington-Hqll, J., Higgs, R. and Edmonds, P. (2005) The healthcare needs of chronic obstructive pulmonary disease patients in the last year of life. *Palliative Medicine*, 19(6), 485–91.

Gold Standards Framework (2009) *Prognostic Indicator Guidance*. http://www.goldstandardsframework.nhs.uk/TheGSFToolkit/Identify/TheThreeTriggers.htm. Accessed: 05 October 2009.

McCarthy, M., Addington-Hall, J. and Altmann, D. (1997) The experience of dying with dementia: a retrospective study. *International Journal of Geriatric Psychiatry*, **12**, 404–9. Cited in: Social Care Institute for Excellence and National Institute for Health and Clinical Excellence (2007) *Guidelines on Supporting People with Dementia and Their Carers in Health and Social Care*. National Clinical Practice Guideline Number 42. British Psychological Society and Gaskell, London.

McGavigan, A. and Dunn, F. G. (2005) Palliative medicine for patients with end stage heart disease. In: *Oxford Textbook of Palliative Medicine* (eds. D. Doyle, G. Hanks, N. Cherney and K. Calman), 3rd edn. Oxford University Press, Oxford.

National Institute for Clinical Excellence (2005) *Chronic Heart Failure: Management of Chronic Heart Failure in Adults in Primary and Secondary Care*. NICE, London.

National Service Frameworks (2000) *Coronary Heart Disease*. Department of Health, London.

National Service Framework (2009) http://www.ucl.ac.uk/dementia/research/nsf.htm. Accessed: 11 October 2009.

National Dementia Strategy (2009) http://www.dh.gov.uk/en/SocialCare/Deliveringadultsocialcare/Olderpeople/NationalDementiaStrategy/index.htm. Accessed 11 October 2009.

Royal College of Physicians (2007) *Palliative Care Services: Meeting the Needs of Patients*. Report of a Working Party. http://www.rcplondon.ac.uk/pubs/contents/ec579e02-64fd-4f36-bb5d-5159a276077f.pdf. Accessed 16 November 2009.

Social Care Institute for Excellence and National Institute for Health and Clinical Excellence (2007) *Guidelines on Supporting People with Dementia and Their Carers in Health and Social Care*. National Clinical Practice Guideline Number 42. British Psychological Society and Gaskell, London.

Waterlow, J. (2009) *Pressure Area Risk Assessment Tool*. http://www.judy-waterlow.co.uk/. Accessed: 11 October 2009.

Zwakhalen, S. M. G., Hamers, J. P. H., Abu-Saad, H. H. and Berger, M. P. F. (2006) Pain in elderly people with severe dementia: a systematic review of behavioural pain assessment tools. *BMC Geriatrics*, **6**. Available at: http://www.biomedcentral.com/1471-2318/6/3.

🖳 Useful websites

British Heart Foundation
http://www.bhf.org.uk/

National Service Framework Document on Coronary Heart Disease
http://www.publications.doh.gov.uk/pdfs/chdnsf.pdf

Patient UK – Respiratory disease information
http://www.patient.co.uk/leaflets/disease_of_lung.htm

National Dementia Strategy
http://www.dh.gov.uk/en/SocialCare/Deliveringadultsocialcare/Olderpeople/
NationalDementiaStrategy/index.htm

National Multiple Sclerosis Society
http://www.nationalmssociety.org/index.aspx

Multiple Sclerosis Society
http://www.mssociety.org.uk/

Motor Neurone Disease Association
http://www.mndassociation.org/

NICE Guidance on Dementia care
http://www.nice.org.uk/Guidance/CG42

Judy Waterlow Pressure Risk Assessment Tool
http://www.judy-waterlow.co.uk/

📋 Chapter links to the Nursing and Midwifery Council Standards of Conduct, Performance and Ethics for Nurses and Midwives (2008)

Section 1: Make the care of people your first concern, treating them as individuals and respecting their dignity

Treat people as individuals
- You must treat people as individuals and respect their dignity
- You must not discriminate in any way against those in your care
- You must treat people kindly and considerately
- You must act as an advocate for those in your care, helping them to access relevant health and social care, information and support

Collaborate with those in your care
- You must listen to the people in your care and respond to their concerns and preferences
- You must support people in caring for themselves to improve and maintain their health
- You must recognise and respect the contribution that people make to their own care and wellbeing
- You must make arrangements to meet people's language and communication needs
- You must share with people, in a way they can understand, the information they want or need to know about their health

Ensure you gain consent
- You must ensure that you gain consent before you begin any treatment or care
- You must respect and support people's rights to accept or decline treatment and care
- You must uphold people's rights to be fully involved in decisions about their care
- You must be aware of the legislation regarding mental capacity, ensuring that people who lack capacity remain at the centre of decision making and are fully safeguarded
- You must be able to demonstrate that you have acted in someone's best interests if you have provided care in an emergency

Work effectively as part of a team
- You must work cooperatively within teams and respect the skills, expertise and contributions of your colleagues
- You must be willing to share your skills and experience for the benefit of your colleagues
- You must consult and take advice from colleagues when appropriate
- You must make a referral to another practitioner when it is in the best interests of someone in your care

Use the best available evidence
- You must deliver care based on the best available evidence or best practice
- You must ensure any advice you give is evidence based if you are suggesting healthcare products or services
- You must ensure that the use of complementary or alternative therapies is safe and in the best interests of those in your care

☑ Self-assessment test

1. Which of the following statements about palliative care for all diagnoses is not true?

    A   The current End of Life Care Strategy is geared towards the needs of all dying people

    B   It is likely that hospices will be overrun with people with chronic conditions and will be unable to function

    C   Many people with a chronic illness would not want to go to a hospice anyway

    D   If education about the needs of all dying people is to make a difference then it needs vastly increased funding, otherwise little will change

2. End stage heart failure is characterized by:

    A   Constipation and palpitations

    B   Food cravings and heightened taste

    C   Breathlessness and anxiety

    D   Neuropathic pain and hiccups

3. Chronic obstructive pulmonary disease is a leading cause of morbidity and mortality to the tune of:

    A   13%

    B   30%

    C   24%

    D   42%

4. Some of the most commonly encountered neurodegenerative conditions include:

    A   Addison's disease, CVA

    B   Epstein–Barr syndrome, shingles

    C   Cerebral ataxia, neuralgia

    D   Motor neurone disease, Parkinson's disease

5. Which of the following symptoms is rarely seen in dementia sufferers in the last year of life?

    A   Urinary incontinence

    B   Short-term memory loss

    C   Pain

    D   High blood pressure

Dealing with ethical dilemmas

He was dying of motor neurone disease at only 25 years old. The noise in the ward and his inability to communicate simply mean that he shrieks louder and louder. Pain is radiating from him to the distress of everyone, and we no longer know what to do. We have tried everything as a team and feel helpless confronted with such suffering. It's my choice to be alongside him, and I acknowledge I may be getting in too deep, but I need to try to help.

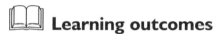

Learning outcomes

After reading this chapter and completing the reflective activities the learner will be able to:

- Understand the core ethical principles that underpin healthcare and professional practise
- Describe the ethical frameworks available that can help in complex ethical decision making
- Reflect on a range of ethical situations encountered that directly affect nursing practice and utilise the good practice guidelines offered

Introduction

As this short clinical anecdote so aptly summarises, there is often a complete sense of powerlessness when confronted by such complex dilemmas. Ethical decision-making is rarely about major life-threatening issues in daily practice, but it is about being treated decently, being listened to, setting acceptable standards and responding to others in a reciprocal way. The young man with MND was receiving the best medical and nursing care available, but his suffering was immense and even the common humanity of the nurses' presence and good communication skills made no difference. Many nurses have encountered such situations in clinical practice and felt completely out of their depth.

I would suggest also that private thoughts surrounding the quality and value of this young man's life are quite common. Such thoughts may not be verbalised, but are nevertheless part of how we reflect and agonise over complex decisions of care that seem insurmountable.

Situations such as this place nurses in a paradox of conflict that pit the societal norms and acceptable ethics and duties of clinical care embodied within codes of conduct and law against the personal views and morality of what is being encountered. In other words the nurse may come to the personal, moral, conclusion that the young man's life is no longer worth living in the face of such suffering and he may be better off dead, but professional, legal and ethical obligations forbid acting on, or even voicing, such concerns.

This chapter will not enter into a detailed debate surrounding the many and complex approaches to ethics, but will concern itself with the main guiding principles that help support the practical reality of behaving ethically with the dying and their family in whatever setting care is delivered.

Ethical principles in healthcare

There are four simple ethical principles which need to be understood when considering the decisions that are made by healthcare professionals about end of life issues. The codes of conduct and guidelines for practice that exist for many professions, including nursing, are underpinned by these four principles, which are (Beauchamp and Childress, 2008):

- **Beneficence**: Doing good for others. The duty to do good and to prevent harm and to act in the best interest of the client.
- **Non-maleficence**: The duty to do no harm. Any intervention needs to be weighed against the good and the bad effects.
- **Justice**: As applied to the person's rights, what the person deserves according to their needs.
- **Autonomy**: The freedom to determine one's own future without external constraints. It relies upon truth telling, accurate information, varying value systems and understanding.

 Reflective activity

Refer to your copy of the Nursing and Midwifery Council's Code of Conduct (NMC, 2008) and cross-reference these principles with a highlighter pen throughout the clauses within the document. You will find many similarities.

What influences ethical decision-making?

Each of us consider ourselves as ethical beings who have a moral stance, values that guide our lives and give us an understanding of right from wrong. We try to apply this knowledge and our life experience into making ethical decisions on a daily basis in even the most simple of life circumstances. Most of the time we get things right, but occasionally we are aware that external factors and previous experiences get in the way of an objective decision and we agonise over what to do. Eventually we make a decision and stand by its consequences. Developing an awareness of these external factors is vital to how we progress through life as mature people and become what many would call 'wise'. It's a lifelong quest and perhaps unachievable, but some of the most important factors include:

Influence	Reactions
The law as we understand it:	Am I free to speak?
Local policies and protocols:	I have to follow procedure
Professional codes of conduct	I have to abide by what it says
Others:	The group I am working with
Past experience:	What did I do last time?
Moral conscience:	Can I live with this decision?
The consequences of my actions:	Have I learnt from past experience?
The influence I have:	I'm only a student
Support from others:	I'm on my own
Culture and religion:	What does my faith say I should do?
Upbringing and education:	What would my parents say?
Energy and drive:	Is it worth the effort?
Relationship to the person(s) or issues:	Should I be loyal to them?

 Reflective activity

Sometimes what is morally wrong in your eyes may be professionally right in clinical practice and you are required to abide accepted codes of practice. For example, the decision of an elderly man to continue smoking has to be respected even though he has been told he will lose his leg unless he stops, as must the decision of a young woman at risk in childbirth of complications to refuse a blood transfusion, if needed, because of her religious convictions.

What principle is being respected here and how would you reconcile yourself to this in clinical practice? Make some notes in your portfolio.

Useful approaches to ethical decisions

There are no easy answers to how we should approach ethical issues, but there are a range of skills and information that can and should be utilised to help. Demonstrating thoroughness in professional practice is not only a moral imperative, so that 'best interest' is served for the patient, but also a legal requirement. Below are some of the main ways in which we can do this.

- **Acknowledgement of our personal beliefs, values, prejudices and feelings**: This is an easy statement to make, but to achieve it requires a high degree of reflective maturity.
- **Involving others**: There is a clear obligation to work collaboratively with other members of the healthcare team where difficult decisions are needed. This is a key component of the NMC Code of Conduct (2008) and essential for informed decision making.
- **Information**: as much as possible from as many sources as possible. Each situation is unique in the context of the circumstances presented; therefore a sound knowledge of such is essential.
- **Standards/protocols**: as well as relevant codes of conduct, local policies should always be referred to for specific advice.
- **Finding out the needs of patients and relatives**: a core component of the palliative approach to care is to find out and respond to the patients' issues as they perceive them.
- **Negotiating skills**: the need for tact, diplomacy, good active listening skills and a non-judgemental, objective approach has never been greater.
- **Humility to learn from our experience**: a willingness to acknowledge our limitations and to actively learn from the rich experiences we encounter, no matter the outcome, and to maintain an intelligent self respect

Some of the key ethical issues in palliative care today

- Collusion to deny the person information
- 'Do not resuscitate' orders
- Advance directives (living wills)

- Hydration close to death
- Sedation close to death
- Assisted suicide
- Double effect – the principle and its validity
- Extraordinary vs. futile treatments
- Withdrawal of treatment
- Hastening death
- Passive/active interventions

This is a daunting list. Many of these situations are rarely encountered in daily clinical practice, yet they achieve a high media profile (e.g. assisted suicide). Others are quite common yet receive little attention either in the media or daily in clinical practice (e.g. collusion) (see Chapter 7 on communication skills for more details on how to handle collusion). This does not diminish their significance, but should in fact guide us towards where our priorities ought to be. Issues such as hydration, sedation and the withdrawal of care are central to good practice with the dying in whatever environment and are rightly beginning to receive much more consideration by policymakers and professional bodies.

Ethical frameworks to help decision making

There are a number of useful well-developed frameworks available to assist in decision making which have been published and evaluated in clinical practice. Perhaps the best known is Seedhouse's ethical grid (1988) (Figure 5.1) which comprises a four-layer grid enabling different aspects of an ethical issue to be worked through in a logical manner.

- The central layer looks at respect, autonomy and the person's needs and is at the core of any decision that is made.
- The second layer, moving outwards, considers deontological (duty) issues such as intent, doing good, minimising harm and truth telling.
- The third layer considers consequentialist issues (the consequences of an action) and asks how this will benefit the individual, a group of people in similar circumstances, and society.
- The fourth layer considers the external forces influencing care, such as those listed earlier.

Each of these layers is seen as independent, yet all clearly have a strong relationship to each other and decision making can move between one layer

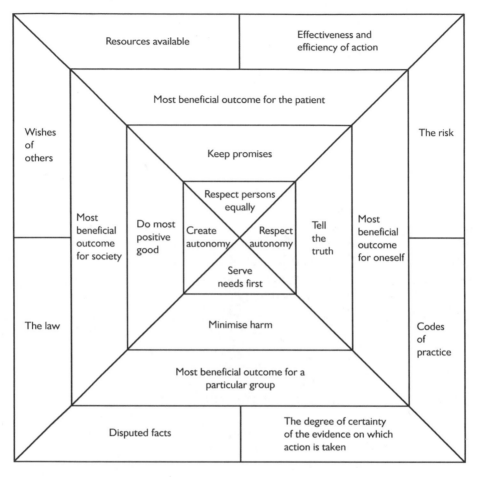

Figure 5.1 Seedhouse's ethical grid (1988).

and another. Its appeal is in its visual representation and its consideration of external forces.

Another approach is Greipp's model (1992) which was developed to take account of the complex social, legal and economic factors which affect health-care decisions today. This model places the same core ethical principles centrally and puts nursing and patient influences on either side. It emphasises the importance of existing knowledge, culture, education and our own personal beliefs on our professional practice. It could be argued that this perspective on ethical decision-making is more in tune with contemporary nursing practice in that it more closely recognises everyday realities.

Niebuhr's model, however, which was developed as far back as the 1960s, brings in the element of intuition to ethical decisions and in the context of palliative care would seem entirely appropriate (Niebuhr, 1963). This model asks the reader to work through a problem by answering a series of questions.

- What is happening now? (based on your gut feeling)
- What would happen if? (certain actions were taken)
- After careful thought what is the most appropriate answer?
- What has been the end result of this action?

The simplicity of this approach is appealing to many particularly as it embraces the abstract element of intuition that is so cherished by nurses in practice. There is still a need to consider the four core ethical principles discussed at the beginning of the chapter and to bring in the influences of professional codes and duty.

No single model will suit all occasions and to offer specific advice on each possible scenario encountered would be impossible, but the important link between ethics and caring has to be the central focus of any decisions made in ethical situations. In this regard it can be argued that nurses have a distinct advantage in that, whilst nursing does not have a monopoly on caring approaches, it is the single most important underpinning principle that defines the profession itself.

The principle of double effect

One of the most controversial and frequently misunderstood aspects of pain control in terminal care is the effect that high doses of opiates have on the patient close to death. There is an increasing body of evidence which dispels the popular myth that respiratory depression is an inevitable consequence of opiate usage in the terminally ill (Bercovitch *et al.*, 1999; Morita *et al.*, 1996; Fohr, 1998). Unfortunately this stance is used all too often by inexperienced doctors and nurses worried about the possible consequences of hastening a patient's death to justify not prescribing appropriate doses of major opiates titrated carefully to the patients' needs. The consequences for the patient are that their pain remains uncontrolled up to the moment of death, and that cannot be ethically justified when the means for relieving distress is readily available.

Double effect is a well-established and accepted doctrine in British law (*R v. Adams* 1957) which enables a doctor to safely make a decision regarding the possible effects of drugs he or she may use to help control pain and difficult symptoms as long as the primary intention of the drug prescribed is to relieve distress; hence the term double effect. In simple terms it asks the question 'What is the intention here?'. It also reflects the important moral principles of (a) doing good for your patient and (b) acting in the patient's best interest – both of which are firmly enshrined in the 2008 NMC Code of Conduct (NMC, 2008).

The Mental Capacity Act

The Mental Capacity Act of 2005 (DoH, 2005) has given much greater clarity to the area of advance decision making at the end of life and the Code of Practice issued in 2007 (Department for Constitutional Affairs, 2007) determines the circumstances under which capacity for decision making is valid and the ability for someone to choose another person (an attorney) to make decisions on their behalf if they lose capacity.

Further discussions in this chapter surrounding advance directives, hydration and sedation are all closely linked to the substance of this valuable piece of legislation. It is pertinent therefore to outline the five key principles that underpin the Act.

1. Presumption of capacity: everyone has the right to make their own decisions and their capacity to do is presumed in law unless incapacity is clearly established.
2. There should be support to help people make such decisions. All practical steps should be seen to have been taken to inform the person of their options under a presumption of capacity, unless demonstrated otherwise.
3. People have the right to make decisions that may seem contradictory, unwise and that may put their health at risk.
4. Best interests: decisions made on behalf of a person who lacks capacity must be demonstrated as working in that person's best interest.
5. The person's rights and freedoms should be respected and restricted as little as possible.

⧗ Reflective point

Notice the heavy emphasis on autonomy, which fits with the model of partnership in care and has close parallels to the NMC 2008 code once again. The act is quite clear that capacity is not an absolute concept and will vary according to the prevailing circumstances and over time. Each situation should therefore be treated as unique, and whilst the guidance can help it is the individual's presumed capacity at any one given time that is paramount.

Advance directives

The advance directive is an American concept which has been adapted and used in the UK in a limited way for close to 30 years now. It is based around the very simple idea that a person can leave instructions about their possible medical treatment, in case there comes a time when they are no longer capable of making decisions or of communicating them.

- **What does it do?** Many people fear that, if they become ill, they could face a situation where they may be given too much treatment when there is little or no chance of recovery, or given treatment which would leave them in a condition they could not cope with. An advance directive can show that in the future, under clearly defined circumstances, the person does not want treatment which will help him or her to live longer, such as antibiotics, tube feeding or being kept alive indefinitely on a life support machine. It is important to recognise that advance directives are an entirely separate issue from voluntary euthanasia, and should not be confused with the debate about assisted dying.
- **Is it legally binding?** Yes – an advance directive does now have legal status in UK law as long as it meets the following conditions:
  - The person is mentally able, is not suffering any mental distress and is over 18 when he or she makes the request.
  - The person was fully informed about the nature and consequence of the advance directive at the time he or she made it.
  - The person is clear that the advance directive should apply to all situations or circumstances which arise later.
  - The person is not pressurised or influenced by anyone else when he or she made the decision.
  - The living will has not been changed either verbally or in writing since it was drawn up.
  - The person is now mentally incapable of making any decision because they are unconscious or otherwise unfit.
- **What are the advantages and disadvantages?** When a medical/nursing team is faced with a difficult decision about what treatment or care to give to a patient who is not able to make a decision, an advance directive will helps the team to know what the patient would have wanted if he or she had been conscious. However, the advance directive will still have to be interpreted to make sure that the situation it describes does still apply to the patient. Apart from allowing the patient to control the treatment he or she receives, the advance directive will also gives the patient the opportunity to discuss difficult issues with close family and friends.
- **What do I do if I come across one?** If you should be made aware of an advance directive's existence by a patient or relative then inform the person in charge. The document does not have to kept by a solicitor and can be kept in the patient's notes. All members of the healthcare team should be made aware of its contents and provided the conditions as outlined above are clear it now has legal validity within the boundaries of the Mental Capacity Act (DoH, 2005).

'Do not resuscitate' orders

Few areas of healthcare cause as much confusion amongst nurses as this contentious issue. What is not in question here is a cardiac arrest affecting a previously healthy individual. The law here is clear-cut: they should be treated until it is obvious they cannot survive the arrest and a doctor decides resuscitation measures should cease. The NMC Code of Conduct (2008) endorses this view entirely. What is of concern is what should happen to those people who have a known terminal diagnosis and whose illness is liable to end in early death, where if CPR were attempted it would be likely to seriously affect their remaining quality of life.

In response to growing public and professional concern the Royal College of Nursing and British Medical Association issued a joint statement in 2007 (RCN/BMA, 2007) to offer up-to-date guidance for practitioners. It concludes that:

Guiding principles

- Timely support for patients and people close to them, and effective, sensitive communication are essential.
- Decisions must be based on the individual patient's circumstances and reviewed regularly.
- Sensitive advance discussion should always be encouraged, but not forced.
- Information about CPR and the chances of a successful outcome needs to be realistic.

Issues for consideration with competent adults

- Ensure the patient has access to information about decision making in relation to CPR being offered.
- Senior health professional should initiate sensitive discussion with the patient.
- Respect the patient's wish not to discuss resuscitation

Assess the clinical issues

- Is CPR likely to restart the patient's heart and breathing?

- Would restarting the patient's heart and breathing provide any benefit?
- Do the expected benefits outweigh the potential burdens of treatment?

Seek consensus

- Responsibility for the decision rests with the consultant or GP in charge of care.
- Record patient's wishes clearly in notes and communicate the decision to relevant health professionals.

Issues for consideration with adults lacking capacity

- Is there a valid and applicable advance refusal of CPR? Yes or no?

Proxy decision makers (Scotland only)

- Consult any appointed proxy decision maker and follow procedures in Adults with Incapacity (Scotland) Act 2000.

Assess the best interests of the patient

- What is known about the patient's wishes regarding resuscitation?
- Did the patient request confidentiality?
- Did the patient identify people to be consulted about treatment?
- Seek the views of people close to the patient about what he or she would want.
- Discuss with the clinical team.

The assessment of clinical issues remains the same as with competent adults. The priorities for nurses working in areas where such issues of resuscitation may be present are to make sure that the local policy is clear, accessible to all, known to all and endorsed actively by the resident medical staff at all levels. It is not acceptable for them to abrogate responsibility for this to either nurses or junior staff because it is too difficult or sensitive an issue.

Careful but assertive diplomacy is required by nurses, who have a professional duty to make sure that patients, family, other nurses and above all the medical staff and area management are all in agreement about what is and is not acceptable.

Euthanasia

For reasons of clarity it would be useful to list the most commonly accepted definitions of euthanasia, assisted suicide and the other terms that are often used in conjunction with these and which potentially cause confusion.

- **Assisted suicide**: Helping a person to end his or her life by request in order to end suffering. (Currently only lawful in Switzerland, where the reasons must be altruistic.)
- **Physician-assisted suicide**: A medical doctor helping the patient to die by prescribing a lethal overdose of appropriate drugs. The patient can choose whether to drink it. (Lawful only in Oregon USA, Switzerland, Netherlands and Belgium.)
- **Euthanasia**: A broad, generic term meaning 'help with a good death'.
- **Voluntary euthanasia**: Death by lethal injection by doctor when requested by patient. (Only lawful in Belgium and the Netherlands for the terminally ill.)
- **Non-voluntary euthanasia**: By using powerful drugs, a doctor ends the life of a dying patient against their will. (Illegal in all countries around the world.)

The act of intentionally ending another person's life by medical assistance is perhaps the most emotive, misunderstood and controversial of all the ethical issues to be faced in healthcare today. With both public and professionals alike this subject raises an immensely complex set of arguments which embrace society's core values and potentially its future laws. It is for this reason that it is hotly debated in the media and continually discussed by professionals. We all have a vested interest therefore in getting it right, because decisions regarding our own health and welfare in future years may well rest on how society views purposeful and deliberate medical assistance to end life, or provision of the means for someone to end their own life.

There are numerous definitions of euthanasia, which in many ways only serve to add to the confusion, but however it is defined the key moral and ethical issues are:

(a) The intention or motive behind the act itself and
(b) The consequences for that individual and society as a whole.

This chapter will not enter into a debate around these issues, nor concern itself with the rapidly changing international scene, but will simply attempt to give an overview of the current legal and ethical advice that is available.

The position for all healthcare staff regarding euthanasia is abundantly clear in British law. Even though they may morally sympathise with a patient's wishes to die and be witness to physical suffering that cannot be fully controlled by modern pharmacological intervention, they are prohibited by criminal law from taking any steps or giving any advice to the patient, or indeed the relatives, to help them carry out that wish (Dimond, 2008).

The principles of euthanasia are based on the assumption that some people, because of their circumstances, are 'better off dead', and their lives are 'not worth living', and also that we should treat them in the same way as we would treat a sick animal. That principle pays no heed to whether the death is voluntary or involuntary. British law is founded on the idea that all human life has equal value and is entitled to protection. It is argued that were a euthanasia law in place it would undermine this latter principle. In other words, to agree that some people, albeit in difficult circumstances, have the right to ask others to assist them to die (even when the other person concerned agrees) they are better off dead, is not accepted in British law.

The RCN the BMA have both issued advice on this subject to help, and copies of the relevant documents can be found on the websites listed at the end of the chapter. There is little empirically gained advice of a pragmatic nature, however, within the abundance of literature that has been written on this subject. Two authors that do attempt to offer advice are Voigt (1995) and Cole (1993), and much of it is of relevance to nurses. Both articles are based on the authors' work with HIV patients and despite the age of the articles they are as relevant today as when they were written.

Cole (1993) cites four case studies which demonstrate widely varying reasons for requesting euthanasia and attempts to give caregivers some ideas about how to respond to these requests. To do so he considers that they need to suspend their own feelings about the morality of a request for euthanasia and be able to acknowledge the reality of the pain that has led a patient to ask to die. The advice offered is to:

- Ask the patient about it
- Acknowledge the request as sincere
- Investigate the reasons behind it
- Correct the correctable, i.e. difficult symptoms, psychological support
- Return control to the patient, i.e. help them to make their own informed decisions
- Think about the spiritual dimension: do they have a faith, or wish to discuss their life?
- Admit your own powerlessness

Voigt (1995) adopts a similar stance, but proposes his own systematic strategy, i.e.

- Determining the patient's fears
- Evaluating the risk of depression
- Determining expectations
- Establishing support networks
- Discussing the options and plans available

Neither author offers a definitive solution and both rightly point out the need for an individualistic approach which is patient-centred. There have been seven attempts since the Second World War to obtain legislation legalising euthanasia in this country, and each time the proposed bill has been overwhelmingly defeated in parliament at the first vote.

Assisted suicide

This issue was last debated in 2005 when Lord Joffey introduced his Assisted Dying Bill (Joffey, 2004). Currently the law on assisted suicide in the UK is also under scrutiny and the Director of Public Prosecution has for the first time been asked to produce clear guidance for the courts on the circumstances under which a person may or may not be prosecuted for assisting some ones death. Those guidelines were published in 2009 (*The Times*, 2009) and read as follows:

Factors likely to lead to prosecution
- Victim did not indicate unequivocally to the suspect that he/she wished to commit suicide
- Victim did not ask personally on his/her own initiative for suspect's help
- Victim did not have a terminal illness, severe and incurable physical disability or severe degenerative physical condition with no cure
- Suspect was not wholly motivated by compassion and stood to gain in some way
- Suspected persuaded, pressured or maliciously encouraged the victim to commit suicide; exercised improper influence and did not take steps to see that others had not
- Victim was physically able to undertake the act of help him or herself
- Suspect was unknown to the victim and gave specific information – e.g. via a website or publication
- Suspect was paid to help the victim

- Suspect was member of an organisation or group with the purpose to providing a physical environment to allow others to commit suicide

Factors against prosecution
- Victim had 'clear, settled and informed wish' to commit suicide
- Victim indicated unequivocally to the suspect that he or she wished to commit suicide
- Victim asked personally on his or her own initiative for the assistance of the suspect
- Victim had terminal illness, severe and incurable physical disability or severe degenerative physical condition for which there was no cure
- Suspect was wholly motivated by compassion
- Suspect was spouse, partner, close relative or close personal friend of the victim, within the context of a long-term and supportive relationship
- Actions of the suspect were only of minor assistance or influence or the help provided was as a consequence of their usual lawful employment
- Victim was physically unable to undertake the act that amounted to 'help' in committing suicide
- Suspect had sought to dissuade victim
- Victim had tried before to commit suicide

This is the first time since the Suicide Act was passed in the 1960s that the law in this area has been clarified and it has only come about due to pressure from the media generated by several high-profile cases of severely ill people travelling to the Dignitas assisted suicide centre in Switzerland.

Reflective point

Note the extensive use of the words 'victim' and 'suspect' which have distinct connotations towards criminality. No doubt the intention is to emphasise that assisted suicide remains illegal within the UK and that the law has not been changed, merely made clearer. Note also the use of the phrase 'severe and incurable physical disability' when listing the conditions that are acceptable regarding non-prosecution. It is suggested that disabled rights groups in the UK will be distinctly worried about such a development, as it implies that their life is of less worth than others and pays no heed to the countless severely disabled people who lead independent fulfilling lives.

The debate as to the efficacy of these guidelines will rage for some time to come and it the first test cases that go through the courts that will determine whether they are of any constructive use to those unfortunate people who feel the need for assistance to end their own lives, and their families who are caught in this moral, ethical and legal minefield.

It is entirely possible that in the near future it is possible that a further attempt at permissive legislation will be forthcoming. There will always be those people in any society that make a conscious and rational decision to end their life. That is a legitimate choice, albeit regrettable. What we as a society have to decide is essentially whether we are prepared to take the risk of passing legislation for that minority to allow others to assist them, potentially at the expense of undermining the care that is offered to the significant majority.

 Reflective activity

How polarised or open are you to the arguments from either the pro-euthanasia lobby or the anti-euthanasia lobby? What are your professional values regarding the value of life? Do you think the law in the UK needs to be changed? Or would that be the start of a 'slippery slope?

Answering such difficult questions is not easy, so the next time you are logged onto the Internet go to the website of a good quality newspaper and in their search engine type in 'euthanasia and assisted suicide' and read about some of the more recent cases that have highlighted these issues. It may help you to be better informed and to gain a balanced opinion in this emotive subject.

The ethics of hydration

There are few subjects in nursing as sensitive as the issue of hydration at the end of life. Nurses have an ethical duty to recognise and treat malnutrition in competent patients as part of optimal care and this is usually attended to by eating and drinking. There is an increasing realisation, however, that artificial hydration of the terminally ill, where it is clearly recognised that the patient is dying and they are not capable of receiving oral nutrition, is not a good idea.

The literature currently demonstrates considerable differences in clinical practice in this area (Bavin, 2007). Some see it as a crucial part of the management strategy, while others see it as an unnecessary burden, believing that allowing natural dehydration rarely causes distress and may in fact be beneficial (Dunphy *et al.*, 1995). There is only a small body of research, and clinical experience appears to provide the basis for most current practice. What common sense tells us, quite clearly, is that where the person is conscious and requesting fluids these should never be denied. Conversely, where the person is slipping in and out of consciousness and the team agree that death may occur within the next few hours or days, hydrating a patient artificially by any means can have a negative and burdensome effect on quality of life.

Allowing natural dehydration can therefore be seen as a normal part of the dying process. There are many instances when patients who are dying choose to give up eating and drinking as they become weaker. The logic against artificial hydration relates to simple physiology. Putting fluids artificially into a body that is slowly closing down means that the kidneys will not be able to process that fluid. There is only one place therefore, for that fluid to go and that is the lungs, with the consequent effects of peripheral or pulmonary oedema and dyspnoea.

The ethical position

We need to remember that a competent patient has the right to refuse artificial hydration, even if it may be considered of clinical benefit to them. Incompetent patients retain this right through a valid advance directive. Allowing natural dehydration to occur at the end of life and actively resisting artificial hydration, where appropriate, is not synonymous with an active intent to end life and influences neither survival nor symptom control.

Guidelines for good nursing practice

- Early discussion with the patient and family to determine the patients' wishes.
- Establish whether the patient has an advance directive. This may provide clear guidance to help decision making and has legal validity now in the UK.
- Always present facts carefully, explain fully the benefits and burdens.
- Ensure excellent holistic care is given at all times.
- Start discussion early, where possible, with the patient and family to determine the patient's wishes.
- Reassure the patient and family that at all times the comfort of the patient is paramount and that that stopping IV/subcut/nasogastric/gastrostomy fluids is not stopping care.
- Where dehydration results from a potentially correctable cause (e.g. over-treatment with diuretics, recurrent vomiting, diarrhoea or hypercalcaemia), artificial hydration may be a valid option in the short term.
- Decisions about whether to hydrate artificially or not should be judged on a day-to-day basis, weighing up the potential harms and benefits.
- Essential comfort measures: give regular mouth care, offer ice cubes and sips of water if tolerated. Provide cream for lips to prevent cracking and encourage the family where appropriate to help provide this care.
- Give good pressure area care, keep the patient clean and dry at all times.

- Listen and support the patient at all times.
- **Remember**: We must be tactfully resistant to sacrificing the interests of the patient to the emotional distress of the relatives.

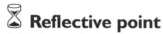 Reflective point

A blanket policy in any clinical area of artificial hydration, or of no artificial hydration, is ethically indefensible. The evidence now against artificial hydration where the person is close to death is compelling. We have readily available clear and useful guidance from the National Council for Palliative Care (NCHSPCS, 2007) and where this is sensitively applied the dignity and comfort of the dying is quite clearly enhanced and we can be confident in our practice (Becker, 2008).

Overall it is likely that patients and relatives will increasingly expect good nutritional care as part of medical treatment to prolong life and improve quality of life: this is their right. It is also likely that the public will increasingly come to accept that hydration or nutrition via a tube should not be used when it impairs the dignity and comfort of those who are dying.

The challenge of palliative sedation

Sedation at the end of life is one area that is immensely sensitive for all health-care professionals, not least for its purported link to hastening death. Research cited below would seem to actively refute that notion and it is important that nurses understand the ethical and professional evidence where sedation is being considered as an active treatment.

Beel *et al.* (2002) conducted a systematic review of the literature in this area and discovered that there was a lot of confusion and inconsistency related to the conceptual definitions of the term 'terminal sedation'. There were also disagreements among many medical staff over the clinical indications for its use alongside inconsistency in pharmacological approaches. Recommendations were that much more qualitative research examining the contextual factors and processes influencing the attitude and behaviour of health professionals and family members is needed.

Defining palliative sedation

the intentional administration of sedative drugs in dosages and combinations required to reduce the consciousness of a terminal patient as much as necessary to adequately relieve one or more refractory symptoms (Broeckaert and Olarte, 2002)

This statement is fully compatible with all current definitions of palliative care which emphasise quality of life and the relief of symptoms where there is unendurable distress, and leaves open the possibility that sedation may be light or heavy, constant, periodic or temporary.

The main clinical indicators for palliative sedation are where there are what are termed *unendurable* and *refractory* symptoms. These include (Ventafridda *et al.*, 1990; Cherny and Portnoy, 1994; Chater *et al.*, 1998):

- Uncontrolled pain
- Respiratory distress
- Delirium
- Nausea and vomiting
- Terminal agitation and restlessness
- Psychological and/or spiritual distress

The meanings of *unendurable* and *refractory* are:

- **Unendurable**: as defined by the patient in both a physical and psychological context
- **Refractory**: symptoms that are intractable and unresponsive to conventional approaches

Other clinical indicators not discussed much in the literature may include palliative emergencies such as uncontrolled seizures, haemorrhage, superior vena cava obstruction, severe acute stridor and multifocal myoclonus. Sedation may also be appropriate for existential distress – 'pain of the soul'. This remains controversial, but should not be ruled out. Much distress is not physical, but mental in its origin and is just as debilitating.

The incidence of refractory symptoms

- 16% hospice patients (Fainsinger *et al.*, 1991)
- 26% hospital patients (Stone *et al.*, 1997)
- 36% in the last 48 hrs (Lichter and Hunt, 1990)
- 48% hospice patients (Morita *et al.*, 1996)
- 50% hospital patients (Braun *et al.*, 2000)
- 52.5% unendurable symptoms (Ventafridda *et al.*, 1990)

The differences in percentages are due to the different approaches in either acute generalist environments or a specialist environment where the incidence of sedation is less. This would indicate that although it is the specialist environment that has the acknowledged expertise to deliver and monitor palliative sedation as an active treatment of choice for patients, it is used less. This may be because of the relative success in the relief of the other elements of the illness (complex pain, existential distress and psychosocial support) and because of this there is a lower incidence of refractory symptoms. Palliative care specialists are perhaps also more comfortable with the concept of sedation, because the ethics of palliative care which centre around a good death are implicit in the care approach.

There are acknowledged limitations in the current research into palliative sedation:

■ Most studies appear to be either surveys of existing practice or empirical observations of practice.
■ We lack understanding of the context of sedation and the human interactions that influence the decision to sedate.
■ Qualitative methodology: grounded theory, clinical ethnography.

Whilst surveys and empirical observation studies are important and have informed us a lot about the nature of what is happening out there, these approaches tend to assume some objectivity and their reliability can be questioned. Interpretations of situations, knowledge of sedation, the context of the environment itself, the social and professional interactions that take place and the highly personal nature of the decision to sedate are all variables that can affect such studies.

The drugs most commonly used for palliative sedation

■ Benzodiazepines – midazolam and lorazepam
■ Neuroleptics – haloperidol
■ Barbiturates – phenobarbitol
■ Opiods alone should never be used for sedation
■ Opiods, where prescribed, should be continued alongside the sedative drugs

A comparative view of the mean survival of patients after starting sedation in the terminal phase gives some interesting results:

Porta Sales *et al.* (1999)	3.2 days
Porta Sales (2001)	2.4 days
Fainsinger *et al.* (2000)	2.4 days

Other studies:
Fainsinger (1998)   4 h – 12 days
Menten (2000)   1–18 days

Would these patients have lived longer had they not been sedated? This is the question that brings us back to the doctrine of double effect. The answer would seem to be no – not according to the current evidence.

What is true is that one cannot deny patients sedation where it is a last resort of appropriate choice for patient comfort at the end of life. Controlled studies are of course impossible to do, but there is little doubt that where applied correctly, palliative sedation is an indispensable approach in a significant number of terminal patients.

The evidence in favour of carefully titrated and sensitively judged sedation as a valid symptom control modality is strong. As shown, there is no real evidence that, where correctly judged as appropriate and correctly administered, life is foreshortened. Palliative sedation is not the back door route to euthanasia that the pro-euthanasia lobby likes so much to put forward. We do lack, however, clear guidance from either medical or nursing professional bodies on this. This is perhaps because of the sensitivities of the subject area and the unfortunate connotation with euthanasia that palliative sedation has. It is therefore all the more imperative that clear guidance is forthcoming.

The law and palliative care

There is no single terminal care act on the statute books in the UK that governs how to approach the dying from a legal perspective. Case precedent and history provide the basis for most law concerning end of life issues and with the numerous high profile cases that have made the media headlines over the last few years, the public are becoming much more aware of these issues.

What needs to be remembered is that case law is underpinned by four principles:

■ Treatment cannot be given without consent
■ There is no automatic right to treatment
■ There is no right to active assisted death
■ Intent needs to be clear

Therefore when caring for patients who are terminally ill we must:

■ Make sure that the person is dying and that this is acknowledged by the whole healthcare team
■ Be certain of our motives, be explicit in our explanations, discuss it with the healthcare team, and accurately record it at all stages

Potential issues include:

- The person's understanding of the nature of the treatment
- Their understanding of the purpose and effects of the treatment
- Their ability to retain this information

Conclusion

Being ethical and being human are one and the same thing. We learn about right and wrong, justice, freedom and the value of life (Thiroux, 1980) as we grow up, and as adults we make decisions on a daily basis using these moral values, which are the foundation of our society and the laws we abide by. The big ethical decisions that involve legislation are the province of government and professional bodies. It is for society and its elected officers to decide the way forward regarding emotive and sensitive areas such as euthanasia and assisted suicide. That doesn't make it any easier for nurses, who have to face such questions on occasion in their work, to know how to handle them.

The real test of any civilised society is not only how it deals with the promotion of good health for its citizens, but also how it deals with those who die. The value that society places on life is at the core of our ethical and legal system and it is nurses who must walk this ethical tightrope on a daily basis (Becker, 2009). Ethics is therefore about much more than the big decisions. It is about how we would like to be treated and how valued we feel as a person, and how this is fostered and respected in our healthcare system. An exercise at a conference many years ago asked the audience this question – If I were dying what would I want? The results of this exercise became known as the 'Dying Patient's Bill of Rights' (Barbus, 1975) and the exercise has been repeated with many audiences in recent years, with similar results every time.

- To have my wish to die in a place of my own choosing respected
- The people who care for me and those closest to me to be caring, sensitive, skilled and honest
  They will demonstrate this by:
- Maintaining a sense of hopefulness, even though the goals will be my comfort rather than my cure
- Explaining things to me tactfully, with sensitivity and in terms I can understand
- Involving me in decisions about my care
- Respecting my need for dignity, privacy and spiritual support

- Allowing me to express my feelings and emotions about my approaching death in my own time and in my own way
- Ensuring that I am free from pain and discomfort
- Treating me with respect, before and after my death
- Comforting me and my loved ones through:
  - their professional counselling skills
  - their use of human senses, such as touch, as and when I appear to need it
  - ensuring that if my loved ones cannot be with me, I will not be left to die alone
  - feeling able to grieve for me when I am gone

This is the closest we can get to an ethical charter for the dying and its relevance lies in the simple act of self-reflection. The rationale is: if this is the standard of care I would like to receive if I were dying, then by default it ought to be close to the standard I expect to deliver for the patients in my care. There is no better arbiter of ethical behaviour and standards than putting oneself into the shoes of the patient.

 Reflective activity

Are there any more items you could add to this list? What would *you* consider important for *you*. Try to include in your list the small but personal things that would add quality to your life, e.g. music, good food, or having a trusted friend nearby.

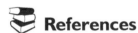 **References**

Adults with Incapacity (Scotland) Act 2000. HMSO, London.

Barbus, A. J. (1975)The dying patient's Bill of Rights. Cited in Ferrell, R. and Coyle, N. (2002) An overview of palliative nursing care. *American Journal of Nursing*, **2**(5), 26–31.

Bavin, I. (2007) Artificial rehydration in palliative care: is it beneficial? *International Journal of Palliative Nursing*, **13**(9), 445–9.

Becker, R. (2008) Providing hydration at the end of life: ethics and practice. Nursing Care Home Supplement. *Nursing Times*, **14**(9), 9.

Becker, R. (2009) Nursing practice commentary: the real test of society is how it deals with dying people. *Nursing Times*, **15**(3), 11.

Beel, A., McClement, S. and, Harlos, M. (2002) Palliative sedation therapy: a review of definitions and usage. *International Journal of Palliative Nursing*, **8**(4), 190–9.

Broeckaert, B. and Olarte, J. (2002) Sedation in palliative care: facts and concepts. In: *The Ethics of Palliative Care: European Perspectives* (eds. H. T. Have and D. Clark). Open University Press, Buckingham.

Beauchamp, T. L. and Childress, J. F. (2008) *Principles of Biomedical Ethics*, 6th edn. Oxford University Press, New York.

Bercovitch, M., Waller, A. and Adunsky, A. (1999) High dose morphine use in the hospice setting: a database survey of patient characteristics and effect on life expectancy. *Cancer*, **86**, 871–7.

Braun, T., Hagen, N., Wasylenko, E., Labrie, M. and Wolsh, G. (2000) Sedation for intractable symptoms of palliative care: do CPGs improve care? Abstract, *13th International Congress on Care of the Terminally Ill*, September 2000, Montreal, Canada; *Journal of Palliative Care*, **16**(3), 88.

Royal College of Nursing and British Medical Association (2007) *Decisions Relating to Cardiopulmonary Resuscitation: A Joint Statement from the British Medical Association, the Resuscitation Council (UK) and the Royal College of Nursing*. RCN, London.

Chater, S., Viola, R., Paterson, J. and Jarvis, V. (1998) Sedation for intractable distress in the dying: a survey of experts. *Journal of Palliative Medicine*, **12**(4), 255–269.

Cherny, N. I. and Portnoy, R. K. (1994) Sedation in the management of refractory symptoms: guidelines for evaluation and treatment. *Journal of Palliative Care*, **10**(2), 31–8.

Cole, R. M. (1993) Communicating with people who request euthanasia. *Palliative Medicine*, **7**, 139–43.

Department for Constitutional Affairs (2007) *Mental Capacity Act 2005 Code of Practice*. Stationery Office, London.

Department of Health (2005) *The Mental Capacity Act*. Department of Health, London.

Dimond, B. (2008) *Legal Aspects of Nursing*, 5th edn. Longman, London.

Dunphy, K. *et al.* (1995) Rehydration in palliative care: if not – why not? *Palliative Medicine*, **9**, 221–8.

Fainsinger, R. (1998) Use of sedation by a hospital palliative care support team. *Journal of Palliative Care*, **14**(1), 51–4.

Fohr, S. A. (1998) The double effect of pain medication: separating myth from reality. *Journal Palliative Medicine*, **1**(4), 315–28.

Greipp, M. (1992) Greipp's model of ethical decision making. *Journal of Advanced Nursing*, **17**(6), 734–8.

Joffey, J. (2004) *Assisted Dying for the Terminally Ill Bill*. HMSO, London.

Lichter, I. and Hunt, E. (1990) The last 48 hours of life. *Journal of Palliative Care*, **6**(4), 7–15.

Menten, J. (2000) *Geocontrollleerde Sedatie: een Therapeutische Mogelijkheid voor Refractaire Symptomen bij de Terminale Paliatieve Patient*. KU Leuven, Leuven.

Morita, T., Inoue, S. and Chihara, S. (1996) Sedation for symptom control in Japan: the importance of intermittent use and communication with family members. *Journal of Pain and Symptom Management*, **12**, 32–8.

Niebuhr, H. R. (1963) *The Responsible Self*, Harper & Rowe, San Francisco.

National Council for Palliative Care (2007) *Artificial Nutrition and Hydration - Summary Guidance*. http://www.ncpc.org.uk/publications/pubs_list2.html

Nursing and Midwifery Council (2008) *Standards of Conduct, Performance and Ethics for Nurses and Midwives*. NMC, London.

Porta Sales, J. (2001) Sedation and terminal care. *European Journal of Palliative Care*, **8**(3), 97–100.

Porta Sales, J., Ylla Catala Bore, E., Estibalez, G. *et al.* (1999) Multi-centred trial in sedation of the terminally ill. *Medicina Paliativa*, **6**(4), 153–8.

R v *Adams* (1957) cited in Randall, F. and Downie, R. S. (1996) *Palliative Care Ethics: A Good Companion*, Ch. 4. Oxford University Press, New York.

Seedhouse, D. (1988) *Ethics: the Heart of Health Care*. John Wiley, Chichester.

Stone, P., Phillips, C., Spruyt, O. and Waight, C. (1997) A comparison of the use of sedatives in a hospital support team and in a hospice. *Palliative Medicine*, **11**, 140–4.

Times Online (2009) *In full: factors for and against prosecution.* http://business.times-online.co.uk/tol/business/law/article6845942.ece. Accessed: 16 November 2009.

Thiroux, J. (1980) *Ethics: Theory and Practice*. Glencoe Publishing, Encino, CA.

Voigt, R. F. (1995) Euthanasia and HIV disease: how can physicians respond? *Journal of Palliative Care*, **11**(2), 38–41.

Ventafridda, V., Rapimointi, C., deConno, F., Tamburini, M. and Cassileth, B. R. (1990) Symptom prevalence and control during cancer patients last days of life. *Journal of Palliative Care*, **6**(3), 7–11.

Useful websites

British Medical Association
http://web.bma.org.uk/ap.nsf/Content/__Hub+ethics

MedEthex online
http://griffin.mcphu.edu/MedEthEx/intro.html

The International Association for Hospice and Palliative Care
http://www.hospicecare.com/Ethics/ethics.htm

StopPain.Org
http://www.stoppain.org/palliative_care/ethics.html

BBC Ethics
http://www.bbc.co.uk/religion/ethics/sanctity_life/euthpallcare.shtml

National Hospice Council
http://www.hospice-spc-council.org.uk/

Royal College of Nursing – go to 'Witnessing resuscitation guidelines for nursing staff'
http://www.rcn.org.uk/members/publications/

Chapter links to the Nursing and Midwifery Council Standards of Conduct, Performance and Ethics for Nurses and Midwives (2008)

Section 1: Make the care of people your first concern, treating them as individuals and respecting their dignity

Treat people as individuals
- You must treat people as individuals and respect their dignity
- You must not discriminate in any way against those in your care
- You must treat people kindly and considerately
- You must act as an advocate for those in your care, helping them to access relevant health and social care, information and support

Collaborate with those in your care
- You must listen to the people in your care and respond to their concerns and preferences
- You must support people in caring for themselves to improve and maintain their health
- You must recognise and respect the contribution that people make to their own care and wellbeing
- You must make arrangements to meet people's language and communication needs
- You must share with people, in a way they can understand, the information they want or need to know about their health

Ensure you gain consent
- You must ensure that you gain consent before you begin any treatment or care
- You must respect and support people's rights to accept or decline treatment and care
- You must uphold people's rights to be fully involved in decisions about their care
- You must be aware of the legislation regarding mental capacity, ensuring that people who lack capacity remain at the centre of decision making and are fully safeguarded
- You must be able to demonstrate that you have acted in someone's best interests if you have provided care in an emergency

Section 2: Work with others to protect and promote the health and wellbeing of those in your care, their families and carers, and the wider community

Manage risk
- You must act without delay if you believe that you, a colleague or anyone else may be putting someone at risk
- You must inform someone in authority if you experience problems that prevent you working within this Code or other nationally agreed standards
- You must report your concerns in writing if problems in the environment of care are putting people at risk

Use the best available evidence
- You must deliver care based on the best available evidence or best practice.
- You must ensure any advice you give is evidence based if you are suggesting healthcare products or services
- You must ensure that the use of complementary or alternative therapies is safe and in the best interests of those in your care

Section 3: Be open and honest, act with integrity and uphold the reputation of your profession

Act with integrity
- You must demonstrate a personal and professional commitment to equality and diversity
- You must adhere to the laws of the country in which you are practising

Uphold the reputation of your profession
- You must not use your professional status to promote causes that are not related to health
- You must cooperate with the media only when you can confidently protect the confidential information and dignity of those in your care
- You must uphold the reputation of your profession at all times

☑ Self-assessment test

1. The main ethical principles which guide healthcare decision making include:
   A   Accountability, beneficence, value of life
   B   Democracy, best interest, paternalism
   C   Doing good, maleficence, autonomy
   D   Freedom, justice, responsibility

2. The Mental Capacity Act is primarily about:
   A Enabling medical staff to make decisions on the patient's behalf
   B Empowering the person to make autonomous decisions
   C Protecting health professionals from litigation
   D Helping the family to make decisions when the patient is incapable

3. The withdrawal of artificial feeding through a PEG (Percutaneous Endoscopic Gastrostomy) tube from a patient dying from end stage heart disease who is expected to die within a few days is:
   A Assisted suicide
   B Acceptable ethical practice
   C Active euthanasia
   D Murder

4. Palliative sedation is:
   A A backdoor unofficial means of euthanasia
   B A last resort when nothing else will work
   C A useful way to ease the family's distress around the bedside
   D A valid means of difficult symptom control where carefully titrated to needs

5. Mrs Jones is being cared for in a nursing home and has been slipping in and out of consciousness for the last 24 hours. Her family are at her bedside and ask you to call the doctor so that an IV line with fluids can be put up to hydrate her. Your response should be:
   A Tell them you will contact the doctor and recommend she be admitted to the local hospital
   B Set up an IV infusion ready and call the doctor in
   C Reassure the family that natural dehydration is a normal and expected part of dying
   D Put in a naso-gastric tube and give plain water through the tube

PART 2

Delivering hands-on care

This part is all about being how to use the evidence-based knowledge, skills and behaviours necessary for the delivery of active, hands on care in whatever setting. It focuses on a range of holistic skills covering everything from meeting death for the first time and communication through to emergencies and the vital areas of pain assessment and management.

Together these subject areas combine to enhance and support quality of life for the patient and family and help them to exercise informed choices in care. For the nurses delivering this care these subjects are at the heart of daily clinical practice and will provide them with a baseline of expertise from which to develop a growing confidence and competence in this most sensitive of areas.

CHAPTER 6

Encountering death for the first time

 Sister asked me to sit with this elderly man who was unconscious and dying, because he had no known family. I was 19, on my first ward as a student nurse, and full of macho confidence, but this scared the hell out of me. I sat behind the curtain reading the newspaper wondering what to do next. Eventually I turned to face him and watched his flickering eyes and his changing expressions. I reached over the bed, held his hand and moments later he squeezed my hand hard. I nearly wet myself, but stayed by his side. He died peacefully about 10 minutes later, still holding my hand.

Learning outcomes

After reading this chapter and completing the reflective activities the learner will be able to:

- Recognise the signs of imminent death where it is an expected event
- Understand the range of nursing responsibilities around the bedside of someone who is dying
- Reflect on the need to access support when dealing with death for the first time

Introduction

There are some events in life that are truly formative experiences. Events that have a profound impact on us and can shape our values, attitudes and beliefs for the future. Being at the bedside of someone who is dying and being surrounded by the intensity of emotions, thoughts and behaviours exhibited is one such life experience. Its impact on a nurse meeting this for the first time can be profound and the memory remains fresh for a long time.

If you would like to test this statement then please take up this small challenge. The next time you go on duty and the moment is appropriate ask an experienced nurse to recall when she was first introduced to death in the clinical situation. You are likely to hear a story in such detail that it might have occurred the previous week, rather than perhaps a decade or two ago. Reflective memories such as this are immensely powerful and can serve as useful learning tool for others.

Where and how do people die?

As a student nurse you will encounter a range of deaths in many different circumstances. However, the vast majority are likely to be expected deaths. The demographics of where and how people die in relation to age profile, cause of death and place of death have changed radically over the course of the past century. Around half a million people die in England each year, of which almost two thirds are aged over 75. Around the year 1900 most people died in their own homes. At that time acute infections were a much more common cause of death and a far higher proportion of all deaths occurred in childhood or early adult life.

The large majority of deaths at the start of the 21st century follow a period of chronic illness such as heart disease, cancer, stroke, chronic respiratory disease, neurological disease or dementia. Most deaths (58%) occur in NHS hospitals, with around 18% occurring at home, 17% in care homes, 4% in hospices and 3% elsewhere (DoH, 2008a).

What happens?

There are many physical changes in the dying process which are quite normal and usually do not cause discomfort: dying patients will manifest some or all of the following:

- Profound weakness
- Difficulty swallowing (e.g. medications)
- The skin may turn pale, darker, blue, purple, patchy – due to peripheral cyanosis
- The body temperature may fall or (in some cases) rise
- Blood pressure is lower and may be harder to hear

- The sensation of being cold or hot may be lost
- Appetite may be lost
- The eyes may glaze over, not blink, stay open, or not see
- The mouth may be dry
- Urine flow may stop or be dark
- Control of bowels and bladder may be lost
- Breathing may become irregular
- Fluid in the lungs may cause a snoring type sound
- There may be more sleepiness and weakness (cannot speak or raise the hand)
- The sense of hearing (and possibly touch) are the last to go

Death itself is usually peaceful, not loud or violent, and it is common for the person to be unconscious in the lead-up to death itself. Often profound skin pallor develops within about half an hour of death. Death is evident when there is no pulse, blood pressure, breathing and brain function for several minutes, and the pupils of the eyes stay wide open and do not change.

How can I help? Your responsibilities

Some of the key nursing strategies that can be used to support patients and relatives when death is imminent are discussed by Becker (2007) and include the following.

Spend time with dying patients

It is all too easy to avoid the dying patient and their relatives. Sometimes they need to be left alone, but there are many times when the need for human contact, comfort and reassurance is vital (Mullard, 2005). The caring concept of 'being available' and 'presencing' is acknowledged by a number of authors. It is synonymous with Parse's (1992) concept of 'true presence' and is one of the carative factors used by Watson (1994). Benner and Wrubel (1989) note that: 'The ability to presence oneself, to be with a patient in a way that acknowledges your shared humanity, is the basis of nursing as a caring practice'.

There will always be a sense of powerlessness when confronted with death. This is something that no one can change. The real skill is in learning to be comfortable with that powerlessness and using it to help the patient and family. We do this by the sensitive use of what is intuitive and felt, as much as by what is learnt (Benner, 1984).

Respect patients' interpretation of their dignity

As a person's physical condition deteriorates they can experience a diminishing sense of control over their life. A patient-centred care approach aims to encourage greater choice and to treat individuals as people rather than conditions. Let the patient decide what their priorities are and work towards these. The governments' Dignity in Care campaign (DoH, 2006) is specifically designed to enhance such choice and dignity.

Don't build a set of beliefs and values which unconsciously communicate to the patient and family that their loved one's death should represent an ideal. There is no right or wrong way to die and many people die with unfinished business in relationships and personal difficulties which are impossible to influence or change; this does not negate or devalue the care that has been given. There is a need to recognise and accept that sometimes, despite the best efforts of the multi-professional team there will always be a nucleus of people who may choose to reject the help offered to them, or whose needs are immensely complex and who cannot be helped as much as we would want. We must therefore learn to evaluate care based on what we know of the patient's values and beliefs and not our own.

Consider the patient's choice about where they wish to be

Although many patients when asked express a wish to die at home, the reality of care today is that few currently achieve that desire (DoH, 2008b). With the bulk of the population therefore dying in some form of institution, careful attention to the environment can provide good psychological support by creating a milieu that the patient is comfortable with. Some patients may prefer peace and quiet and wish to be in a side room. Others, however, like to be part of life on a ward and feel less isolated within a bay environment. Such choice may not be available within the nursing and residential home, but the opportunity to personalise care within that environment is usually better due to greater continuity in staff and often more long-term relationships. Those that die at home can have a wide variety of services to support them (depending on diagnosis, unfortunately), but the psychological comfort of being in familiar surroundings is a powerful element. The key ideas to consider are choice and forward planning.

Understand the family's needs

It is good practice to assign a member of staff to discover what family and friends there are, how they wish to be involved in care and what, if any, special needs they may have. In hospital environments or care homes this is not only part of admission procedure, but a continuing responsibility thereafter, as relationships change and staff come and go. Although difficult to achieve in some clinical areas, the sense of continuity achieved by this approach is highly valued by both patient and relatives (Becker, 2007).

Good communication: answer questions

The skilled use of communication skills to help build and establish a good working relationship with the patient and family is the first stage in delivering quality care. Much has been written about the specialist nature of such skills when used by advanced practitioners in clinical specialist posts (Skilbeck and Seymour, 2002) but for the practising nurse at the bedside the range of competencies needed are generic in nature and highly effective when used well.

It is essential that information about diagnosis, treatment options and prognosis is communicated with honesty and sensitivity by nurses who have the expertise to do so. Without this, it is much harder for people to take decisions about their care, leaving them disempowered by the advance of their illness.

All members of the direct caring team should have up-to-date knowledge about a patient's condition and should be prepared to share this if requested. There is much anxiety expressed by practising nurses about this area, but there is no code, rule, or law which forbids a nurse to give this information if in their judgement it is the right thing to do at the time. It is a matter for careful judgement in the context of the situation at the time, and accountability for such decisions is enshrined in the Code of Professional Conduct (NMC, 2008). We need to be sensitive, however, to the working relationships we have with our colleagues and to our responsibility to the patient to handle questions with the utmost care. Equally, as nurses, there is a clear responsibility to advise non-professional and junior staff how to deal with questions, and when to seek help.

Support with the practicalities of dying

Guidance and support in accessing benefits and managing financial arrangements, wills and social care needs (including the loan of specialist equipment, for example) is vital and nurses need to know who to contact within their locality to action this. Seek out local policies and literature and keep a list of these available for all in the team. Many patients and family members will have access to the Internet today, so it can be helpful to compile a list of suitable websites where more detailed information can be found. At a time of great stress people desperately and sometimes urgently need specialist help and advice if they are to get what they need, when they need it.

Recognise futility

One of the major challenges of palliative nursing in non-specialist environments is empowering staff to reach a considered decision regarding the care orientation of the patient. Ideally, this should be done in conjunction with the patient (if possible), the relatives and all members of the team. Much distress can be caused if efforts to initiate resuscitation or other procedures are fruitless when the quality of the remaining life is poor (BMA and RCN, 2007). It is the simple ethical principle of 'non-maleficence'; or in other words: we should do the patient no harm. The Nursing and Midwifery Code of Professional Conduct (2008) makes this quite explicit. The whole team should ask themselves whether intravenous infusions, parenteral feeding, and the use of subcutaneous fluids are useful and appropriate. The decision to withdraw such treatment is ethically, morally and legally defensible if the team agrees that it is in the patient's best interest. The family's views should be listened too and acknowledged, but are secondary in this instance.

It requires an assertive and knowledgeable nurse who has a good understanding of accountability and confidence to challenge the status quo where necessary if the patient's best interest is to be served.

Helpful guidelines:

■ Discuss the rationale for the current treatment regime to ensure all staff understand what the care priorities are
■ Talk with the patient to explore the issues raised
■ Reassess the level of pain, symptom control or anxiety about their health status
■ Review the management plan regularly
■ Remember that the focus here is on quality of life

Support for yourself and your colleagues

Being at the bedside of someone who is dying can have a profound impact on a nurse. It is a formative learning experience and can shape our professional values, attitudes and beliefs for the future. For this reason it is vital that we not only know how to find support for ourselves at such difficult times, but we are aware of the needs of the others in the team who may be less experienced and are encountering death for the first time in a professional context. There are five simple principles to remember to guide your practice.

1. **Support**: Tell staff that this is your first experience and ask for help. Problems often occur simply because staff assume that you have experience in this area, either because you appear confident or because you are afraid to ask as you don't wish to appear incompetent. The good news is that your honesty will almost always be rewarded by being mentored by a nurse who is interested and sensitive.
2. **Sensitive**: Be aware that this is a unique occasion and not only will the relatives feel vulnerable, but you also. You are being asked to step into and be part of one of life's most sensitive events. The family and friends around that bedside will consider you the expert, even though you are not. They have a right therefore to a professional and caring approach which embraces both the science and art of palliative nursing, as discussed in Chapter 1. This means that you may well feel upset, and on occasions demonstrate this by shedding a tear, or perhaps hugging a family member. Rest assured that this is no contradiction to professional practice; it does in fact enhance it. See the discussion on intrapersonal skills in Chapter 2.
3. **Talk**: Be sure to find a trusted person to talk to about it afterwards. If you have a mentor or other such person available then use them for this purpose. It is important that your perceptions are shared and shaped in this way, so that good practice can be valued and potential issues addressed early on. If no such person is available at work then seek out a good friend or relative who can give you some quality time soon after.
4. **Alone**: If it is avoidable, no patient should die alone. There are always occasions when this is unavoidable, such as when someone lives alone, or during the night, or even when they are in the toilet in a busy hospital environment. There are numerous times, however, when a death is anticipated and expected. When this is the case no person should, unless they request it, be allowed to die alone. This is a clear nursing responsibility and should be taken seriously wherever dying takes place.
5. **Time**: Give yourself time to reflect on the significance of this event and how it has shaped your thinking. Reflective learning is not only an essential part of professional development; it also allows us to validate and gain a sense of perspective about what took place.

Reflective activity

To gain a better insight into your first encounter with death, please read this short extract from a published clinical article and answer the questions it poses.

James's mouth was partially open, his breathing erratic and laboured. His emaciated and jaundiced face resembled a wax-work figure in the dim light of the side ward. James lay motionless, his body showing vivid signs of the battle he had undergone against his terminal liver cancer. I sat quietly, but not at ease, watching every rise and fall of his chest. James had suffered for many weeks. He had grown close to all the staff in the ward during his illness and had requested to die here as he had no family and his friends lived far away. Tonight it was my turn to try to offer him comfort and support during the long, quiet hours of the night shift. I pondered the meaning and significance of life, which at times seems so unfair. My attention turned to James. What was he feeling as he approached the end of his life? I started to think about my own end. How and when would that happen? I suddenly felt very cold and alone. I was brought back to the present when James's hand gently squeezed mine and he gave a shallow sigh. Then his breathing ceased and he lay still. The expression on his face had changed to one of peace and contentment. Death had visited the side ward not as an enemy, but as a friend.

McSherry, W. (1996) Reflections from a side ward. *Nursing Times*, **92**(33), 29–31.

Questions:
1. Pick out some of the key words and phrases that made an impact on you when reading this story.
2. Now write down a few words or phrases that describe how you personally felt immediately after reading this story.

Consider:
- Was it difficult to write down how you felt?
- How similar was this experience compared to your own?

Conclusion

Working with the dying and bereaved is well recognised as one of the most stressful aspects of healthcare, and particularly so for student nurses (Cooper and Barnett, 2005). Preparing yourself for this kind of work is important, because in the long term the emotional burden can build up and cause health problems.

- Know your patients, their condition and circumstances thoroughly
- Know the patients perception of their situation
- Be confident in your skills both clinically and with people and learn not to be afraid of difficult questions and situations
- Learn the value of presence and good listening

- Know how to use the resources and skills of the other members of the team to help you
- Seek out a friendly supporter and listening ear
- Learn to use this supporter or a more formal network if one is in place
- Accept that sometimes difficult situations can never be changed
- Don't expect people to die in a way that represents your beliefs and values
- Regularly examine your own thoughts and feelings about death and dying. What do these events mean to me? What do I value and believe?

Beverley Harper's research in this area, first published in 1977, still has relevance in today's more complex healthcare environments (Harper, 1977). Her contention was that learning to deal with the issues inherent in such work is often done in stages. These stages are not fixed, and indeed as with most linear models a person can move forwards or backwards depending on the circumstances encountered.

- Stage 1 – Knowledge
  - Getting to grips with the subject area and the issues
- Stage 2 – Trauma
  - Becoming emotionally involved and confronting loss personally
- Stage 3 – Grieving
  - The 'grow or go' stage, where we make a choice to either develop our skills and self-awareness or leave the situation and possibly the job
- Stage 4 – Emotional arrival
  - The point where we feel we are able to offer true empathy in a meaningful way
- Stage 5 – Compassion
  - Empathy combined with maturity and an ability to relate to people with deep compassion

There are many potential sources of stress when caring for the dying and those bereaved, and everyone needs both personal and professional support. Often the more formal systems, such as counsellors and groups, simply don't work as people choose not to use them. The real secret of success is in the clarity of the team ethos and philosophy in the work area, combined with an open, honest and people-centred approach that sees staff support as an integral part of the system of care. It is a simple fact that staff who feel valued in any work environment will be better motivated and will cope with complex situations with more confidence. It is not a luxury, but a reflection of the true value we place on our staff.

References

Becker, R. (2007) Psychosocial dimensions. In *Palliative Nursing: Improving End of Life Care*, 2nd edn (eds. S. Kinghorn and S. Gaines). Baillière-Tindall, Ediinburgh.

Benner, P. (1984) *From Novice to Expert: Excellence and Power in Clinical Practice.* Addison-Wesley, California.

Benner, P. and Wrubel, J. (1989) *The Primacy of Care.* Addison-Wesley, California.

Royal College of Nursing and British Medical Association (2007) *Decisions Relating to Cardiopulmonary Resuscitation: A Joint Statement from the British Medical Association, the Resuscitation Council (UK) and the Royal College of Nursing.* RCN, London.

Cooper, J. and Barnett, M. (2005) Aspects of caring for dying patients which cause anxiety to first year student nurses. *International Journal of Palliative Care Nursing*, **11**(8), 423–30.

Department of Health (2006) *Dignity in Care Campaign.* http://www.dh.gov.uk/en/SocialCare/Socialcarereform/Dignityincare/index.htm. Accessed: 18 February 2009.

Department of Health (2008a) *End of Life Care Strategy – Executive Summary.* DoH, London.

Department of Health (2008b) *End of Life Care Strategy: Promoting High Quality Care for All Adults at the End of Life.* DoH, London.

Harper, B. C. (1977) *Death: The Coping Mechanisms of the Health Professional.* South Eastern University Press.

Mullard, E. (2005) Presencing: the unseen therapeutic relationship. In: *Hidden aspects of Palliative Care* (eds. B. Nyatanga and M. Astley Pepper). Quay Books. Salisbury.

McSherry, W. (1996) Reflections from a side ward. *Nursing Times*, **92**(33), 29–31.

Nursing and Midwifery Council (2008) *Standards of Conduct, Performance and Ethics for Nurses and Midwives.* NMC, London.

Parse, R. (1992) Human becoming: Parse's theory of nursing. *Nursing Science Quarterly*, No. 5, 35–42.

Skilbeck, J. and Seymour, J. (2002) Meeting complex needs: an analysis of Macmillan Nurses' work with patients. *International Journal of Palliative Nursing*, **8**(12), 574–82.

Watson, M. (1994) Psychological care for cancer patients and their families. *Journal of Mental Health*, **3**, 457–65.

✍ Chapter links to the Nursing and Midwifery Council Standards of Conduct, Performance and Ethics for Nurses and Midwives (2008)

Section 1: Make the care of people your first concern, treating them as individuals and respecting their dignity

Treat people as individuals
- You must treat people as individuals and respect their dignity
- You must treat people kindly and considerately
- You must act as an advocate for those in your care, helping them to access relevant health and social care, information and support

Collaborate with those in your care
- You must listen to the people in your care and respond to their concerns and preferences
- You must make arrangements to meet people's language and communication needs
- You must share with people, in a way they can understand, the information they want or need to know about their health

Ensure you gain consent
- You must ensure that you gain consent before you begin any treatment or care
- You must respect and support people's rights to accept or decline treatment and care

Section 2: Work with others to protect and promote the health and wellbeing of those in your care, their families and carers, and the wider community

Share information with your colleagues
- You must keep your colleagues informed when you are sharing the care of others
- You must facilitate students and others to develop their competence
  Work effectively as part of a team
- You must consult and take advice from colleagues when appropriate

Section 3: Provide a high standard of practice and care at all times

Keep your skills and knowledge up to date
- You must recognise and work within the limits of your competence

■ You must take part in appropriate learning and practice activities that maintain and develop your competence and performance

Keep clear and accurate records
■ You must keep clear and accurate records of the discussions you have, the assessments you make, the treatment and medicines you give and how effective these have been

☑ Self-assessment test

1. Which combination of words best reflects the physical changes which occur as part of the dying process?
   A Profound weakness, headaches, high blood pressure
   B Fluctuating consciousness, difficulty swallowing, irregular breathing
   C Flatulence, incontinence, high temperature
   D Pale skin, increased sensation, loss of appetite

2. How can you help to support patients when death is imminent?
   A Allocate the patient a side room and respect the family's privacy thereafter
   B Maintain all life-preserving measures so that the family are reassured
   C Adopt an honest, partnership approach and anticipate needs by allocating key staff
   D Refer the situation to the doctor, social worker and chaplain

3. When encountering death for the first time its important to:
   A Put your emotions on one side and get on with it as sensitively as possible
   B Follow correct policy and procedure to the letter
   C Allow senior staff who have more experience to deal with the situation while you watch
   D Seek the support of another experienced member of staff who can work with you

4. Most people given the choice would prefer to die in hospital where the support services are available. Is this statement:
   A True
   B False

5. One of the greatest fears for dying patients in a busy hospital environment is loneliness and isolation. Is this statement:
   A True
   B False

CHAPTER 7

Communicating with care and compassion

 I lay on my bed, terrified and isolated, watching and listening. I know I have cancer – the consultant told me two weeks ago. It was as if nothing had happened. Nurses dashed past with their busy masks. Doctors towered over me chanting their jargon. Had anyone any idea what I felt like? Did anybody care?

Learning outcomes

After reading this chapter and completing the reflective activities the learner will be able to:

- Describe the core components of a meaningful therapeutic conversation
- Understand the underlying factors that contribute to both successful communication and unsuccessful interactions
- Utilise a range of helping strategies that can be used to enhance communication with the dying and those important to them

Introduction

As the short clinical story above illustrates, good communication in a palliative context is sometimes about the delivery of major life-changing information, but more often it is about the regular daily contact and attention we give our patients and demonstrating that we care about the experience they are going through. Culturally, the 'brave face' is commonplace in many busy clinical situations, so it requires a perceptive nurse with good observational skills to recognise distress beyond the superficial pleasantries that dominate the delivery of hands-on care.

We rarely see ourselves as others see us, and to develop the confidence and insight to be able to alter our behaviour towards others so that we may communicate better with them is perhaps the ultimate goal for any nurse. To do so takes a reflective maturity that some would say only comes with a high level of knowledge and experience. Where does that leave the student nurse who, having attended a series of lectures and presentations focused around the basics of enhancing communication, finds themself at the bedside of a patient who says:

> I think I'm going to die nurse, in fact I'm sure of it, but I'm scared and I can't show my fear to my wife. What can I say to her and can you help me find the right words?

Such incidents are not uncommon, and conventional wisdom would dictate that the student nurse finds a more experienced colleague who could perhaps handle the situation whilst they watch and hopefully learn from a good role model. The reality of clinical practice has no such guarantees, however, and it's important that the theory of the classroom can be translated into practice in an accessible and user-friendly way. It's simply not possible to refer to an article, textbook or teacher's handout at such times, so what's necessary is that the student nurse has a small but usable repertoire of evidence-based communication skills at their fingertips, that can be drawn from memory in an instant and used effectively to facilitate a meaningful conversation. There are no guarantees as to the outcome of such a conversation, but we can say with confidence that when used appropriately these skills will help engender both trust and confidence from the patient.

This chapter will look at the varied components that comprise what we understand as good communication skills in a palliative care context and will offer the reader a range of tried and tested strategies and hints and tips for managing difficult and sensitive scenarios just like the one mentioned above.

Why do we avoid communication with the dying?

- Fear of the unknown situation
- Fear that our lack of knowledge may cause more problems
- Fear of unleashing an emotional reaction
- Fear of being blamed
- Fear that we may get upset

These are genuine, heartfelt concerns and are based around our perception that what happens around the bedside of someone who is dying is so full of emotion that it makes for a very unpredictable situation. Reality is somewhat different, however, because the majority of expected deaths in any environment follow a steady process of decline (see Chapter 6), and whilst emotion is present the family and friends around the bedside work hard at putting on a 'brave face' to those around them. It is also true that saying something wrong and being blamed for making an inappropriate remark is highly unlikely.

Reflective point

Both the dying and those surrounding them know that we find it hard to say the right thing. They experience it themselves and recognise it with others around them, including nursing staff.

Important: If you find it difficult to express yourself and use language that is more colloquial than professional the family will forgive you, but only if you demonstrate in your manner that you care.

Perception

Visual perception is an unreliable means of interpreting messages and there are countless examples of optical illusions that trick the mind into seeing one message interlaced within another. It only takes a short while, however, for the person viewing the illusion to realise their mistake and to adjust their vision to take into account the alternative picture. Even when a group of people visualise the same thing at the same time, perception is unreliable because our life experience, knowledge and expectations of the imagery will cause us to interpret the message differently from others. This can have potentially disastrous consequences in clinical practice. Take for example the elderly, confused, sweating and aggressive man who presents at a health clinic. His conversation is incoherent and his awareness of time, place and person is clearly impaired. To a nurse qualified in mental health the perception may be of a person who is suffering from an as yet unidentified form of psychosis. To an adult nurse experienced in medical care he is showing all the signs of out of control diabetes. To an elderly care nurse he may have a chest infection, urinary tract infection or perhaps even constipation.

Written messages are usually more reliable, but even here there can be little reliability if the language used is open to misinterpretation. I am reminded of the classic line written in many nursing care plans – 'the patient was placed on a fluid balance chart'. To other nurses the meaning may be clear, but to a layperson or legal counsel for a healthcare trust investigating a complaint against a nurse it is yet another example of internal jargon that is meaningless and does not reflect well on the nursing profession.

Auditory messages ought therefore to prove much more reliable, because the message given has a particular context at the time and the receiver can interpret this context quickly and place a clear unambiguous meaning to the message. Unfortunately, this is not the case. Take the example below, which is repeated in hospital or nursing home settings every single day.

> The doctor walks into the room, smiles and asks 'How are you today Mrs Smith?' She looks at him and says 'I'm fine thank you Doctor'. The doctor looks down at his notes and scribbles a few words. He thinks he has gathered relevant clinical facts of her progress to inform her treatment, whilst Mrs Smith thinks she has just been polite to the nice young doctor.

The one minute rule

Whenever we walk into a situation where we are the focus of attention, those around us form an impression of us very quickly. This applies whether we are talking to patients/clients and relatives, conducting a team handover between shifts on a ward, or even teaching at the bedside. Experts in interviewing patients (Smith, 2001) tell us that the first minute will most likely shape that impression in the following ways:

- **55%** Visual: facial expression, eye contact, mannerisms, posture, clothes, hair
- **38%** Voice, tone, inflection, accent
- **7%** Content

Get the 93% represented by the first two items right and you will have the full attention of your audience. The 7% will thereafter grow significantly. The cited figures here are approximate and will vary according to the situation, but not by much. One minute is very little time to communicate effectively and build the foundations of a trusting and therapeutic relationship with our patients, but get this minute wrong and you will find it almost impossible to retrieve the situation later.

You will notice that the visual, non-verbal impression has the highest percentage. Auditory messages come next on the list and by far the smallest percentage is the actual substance of what we say. A lot can be learned from this and it relates directly to our opening discussion in this chapter on perception. We have already acknowledged just how unreliable such perception can be unless the messages delivered are absolutely clear and unambiguous. This makes the first minute in which we meet our patients and their family perhaps the most important of all in our care for them.

It is the small but significant things that matter to the patient and family, such as:

- A clean, well-pressed uniform
- Neat and tidy hair
- An upright posture
- A smile
- Appropriate eye contact respecting gender, age, culture or disability
- A clear introduction of self

and most important of all:

- An attitude that reflects your positive interest in them as a person

Reflective activity

Next time you are on duty and are about to meet a new patient or family member, just before the encounter run through a quick mental check in your mind of the bullet points above and adjust your behaviour and stance accordingly. You may be surprised at the outcome.

Trust

It's impossible to overemphasise the importance of trust when dealing with sensitive situations in a palliative care context, and effective compassionate communication that builds, maintains and cherishes trust is at the very heart of palliative care, whether we are managing pain and difficult symptoms, comforting the bereaved or easing spiritual distress. Ensuring that all involved in the patient's care receive appropriate and timely information and support is enormously complex, requiring attention to detail and commitment. Students of healthcare spend much of their time in direct patient care. Consequently, opportunities to really make a positive contribution to care are always present. The words of Stephen Covey (1989) – 'Seek first to understand, then to be understood' – form a useful foundation for all communication, be it with patients, families or colleagues. Listen carefully, don't be in haste to find a simple solution to complex problems and take every opportunity to communicate effectively. Your patients and their families will thank you for it.

Dunlop (1999) suggests we are literally the patient's servant. We must ask, he believes, 'What is it that you feel you need? I am here as your textbook. Open me at whatever page you feel you think might be helpful'. He goes on to discuss complex questions such as when a patient expresses a wish to end their life. This question *must* be explored because it is usually related to feeling a burden or the early indicators of a clinical depression, or because of pain or other symptoms. The patient deserves an exhaustive search for palliative alternatives, after which some change their minds about wanting to die. Our job is not to ignore such a request, nor to pass it on necessarily to another health professional, but to discuss it. (see Chapter 5 for a useful framework for handling this situation).

For some reading this chapter it may seem daunting to address such fundamental questions about life and death. 'I am only a student', seems a perfectly reasonable excuse. In a short time you will be 'only' a staff nurse, then perhaps 'only' a sister/charge nurse. If you don't have the courage to face issues such as this I guarantee they will not become easier if you leave them until you are 'older and wiser'.

Reflective point

The patient chose you because they trust you. Avoiding the question not only leaves the patient still searching but undermines the trust we try so hard to achieve and are privileged to have. The patient will come more than halfway to meeting us when we first encounter them. Nurses, by virtue of their professionalism and commitment are almost universally regarded as trustworthy people. That is an honour few professions have in the public eye. The onus is therefore on us to use that trust effectively and build on it, by our skilled use of communication skills combined with a mature awareness of self. Please remember that dying people prefer to talk about life rather than death and dying. Most conversations with dying patients are not about death or dying, but we must be ready to 'change gear' if and when necessary.

Does the patient know? Does the patient want to know?

Much pain can unwittingly be caused by staff and relatives who make assumptions about what the patient knows and wants to know about their illness. Patients often have a very good idea about what is wrong with them. Consider Jim, a 68-year-old man who has smoked for almost 50 years. As he chats with his doctor about his worsening chest condition and the new terrifying symptom, haemoptysis, it is very unlikely that the possibility of cancer has not crossed his mind. Finding out what the patient knows *and* wants to know is the key to dealing with this complex issue.

A conversation between Jim and his GP

Jim: This has got me worried this time doctor.

GP: What's going through your mind this time?

Jim: Well you put 2 and 2 together don't you?

GP: Do you want to tell me what you come up with or is that a bit scary?

Jim: It's far too scary!

GP: Are you ready for me to tell you what I have come up with?

Jim: Umm... yes doc, but no gory details, just lay it out on the line...

GP: You're quite sure Jim?

Jim: Go for it, as the kids say these days.

GP: This could be another chest infection or your bronchitis getting worse, but I am more concerned today because of the blood.... Shall I tell you what's on my mind?

Jim: Yes please, I have to know.

GP: Jim there is a strong possibility that you may have lung cancer.... Is that a shock to you?

Jim: Yes and no... I have ignored the warnings on the packets but you always hope you will get away with it.... What's next doc?

The GP then went on to discuss investigations. He offered to talk about treatment options should the diagnosis be confirmed, but Jim declined.

⧗ Reflective point

- Serious illness is not always a complete shock to the person, but is almost always frightening.
- Patients will tell you what they want to know if you allow them to – always offer a choice.
- Use simple language and go at the patient's pace.

For further information about breaking bad news, see Buckman (2005).

Developing our conversations

We may need to ask direct questions about sensitive issues rather than waiting for the patient to ask us. If you find this difficult it may be because you do not want to distress the patient. Alternatively, it may be because you wish to avoid confronting your own pain and fear. Think carefully about this and find someone you trust to talk to. When teaching I regularly encounter students who become upset. When talking with them they will tell me about what has upset them. Often they tell of events in the distant past that they have not confronted. They may decide to discuss such issues with a GP, counsellor or psychologist. Acknowledging and telling the story can be sufficient to resolve what has happened. Others deal with traumatic events by 'filing them away' in the mind and using denial. This is one way of coping, and sometimes an effective way, but be aware that this could have a negative effect on your ability to help patients. If in doubt, seek some confidential advice.

Spending time with patients

Nurses who spent time with patients in the past were often criticised and frequently felt guilty, because the importance of the ward routine and the hands-on tasks took precedence. Times have changed, but old habits and customs change slowly. Nowadays nursing is conducted at a rapid pace with high patient turnover and discharge pressures. We feel that something else is always more important and we must be seen to be doing something. Using the palliative approach effectively is not about sacrificing the vital and important tasks of nursing to sit with a person and engage in life and death conversations to the exclusion of all else. It is more about developing an attitude of mind that is open and sensitive to situations as they develop whilst doing our job.

If you are a student of nursing then your opportunity to engage in such conversations is a daily occurrence. Cross check with your mentor and create an environment where such work is both encouraged and valued.

Caring and compassion will not be perceived by your patients as proportional to the time spent with them. You will be judged by the relationship you develop and your ability to demonstrate respect, compassion, love and understanding.

Listening and attending skills

Paraphrasing consists of putting the patients' words into our own words while *reflecting* indicates that we are trying to understand the patient's feelings. *Summarising* during and towards the end of a conversation allows us to piece together the patient's story and check that we have understood. At times we may need to *challenge* and *confront* a patient's behaviour, although this may sound harsh. Aim for most of your *questions* to be open to allow free-flowing conversation but closed questions have their place when asking factual questions. Two simple questions to ask yourself about your conversations with a patient are, 'Is this nurse or patient centred?' and 'Who is doing most of the talking?'. If it is nurse-centred or you are doing most of the talking think about how you can redress the balance.

Listening is a complex and active process. In essence it requires that we give our full and undivided attention to another person. Sitting down and making gentle eye contact sends the powerful message, 'I am here for you'. In the course of listening we use skills which you will be familiar with.

Active listening is an intentional act, involving a high degree of concentration and effort on the part of the receiver. The skill of listening is not a natural ability; it must be worked at and developed over a period of time. Good active listening almost always increases self-esteem. It is a way of saying to the person 'You are important'. This is why active listening is such a powerful force in carer–client relationships.

Be very aware of your non-verbal communication and where possible set things up to provide the best possible environment. Ask yourself these questions both before and after your encounters:

Posture:
- How did I greet them?
- How did I talk to them?
- Did I sit or stand?
- Could they see my face?
- Were my mannerisms and posture welcoming?

Eye contact:
- Did they seem comfortable?
- Where did I look most?
- Can I look at them when they are speaking to me?

Language:
- Was the tone of my voice friendly?
- Did I speak at their level?
- Do I use prompts or repeat words?

Observation:
- What did I see when I first encountered this person?
- How were they behaving?
- What were their mannerisms telling me?

Privacy:
- Was privacy achievable in the environment?
- Did I do anything to influence this?

Personal space:
- Where did they sit?
- Where did I sit?
- Was the distance safe for the other person?
- Could I have touched them if needed – would it have been appropriate?

Dealing with difficult questions

In *Harry Potter and the Philosopher's Stone* (Rowling, 1997), Dumbledore, the Headmaster, says:

> The truth is a beautiful and a terrible thing and should therefore be treated with great caution. However, I shall answer your questions unless I have a good reason not to, in which case, I beg you to forgive me. I shall not of course tell a lie.

Patients do ask direct questions, but be alert for difficult questions hidden behind a mask. Patients who mask their difficult questions are generally too frightened to ask them outright. Unfortunately they are easy to miss

What makes a question difficult?

- I don't know the answer
- I know the answer but I don't know if I am allowed to tell the patient
- A relative has told me not to tell the patient
- The answer will be hurtful and I am unsure about the consequences of telling the truth

Some examples of openly difficult questions

- How long have I got?
- Does this mean the cancer has come back?
- What will it be like?

- You won't let me die in pain will you?
- Have I got cancer?
- Am I going to die?
- Will you put me out of my misery?

Some examples of 'masked' difficult questions

- I seem to be losing so much weight, I wonder what that can be?
- Do you get many patients in here with this?
- My uncle had something like this and, well, he...
- These tablets don't seem to be making any difference do they?
- I wonder how John will cope in the future.

All these questions are difficult because either we do not know the answer or the answer will cause pain and distress. A difficult question should be the stimulus for a dialogue and not merely something that requires a simple answer.

When a patients asks us difficult question they have usually thought long and hard and chosen someone they can trust. They expect from us an honest response demonstrating that we understand and wish to help. Often we will not know the full answer, including all the clinical details. It is not a failing to admit this. If we try to bluff our way out we will be discovered and we will destroy trust.

Giving information

Patients need information, but they need intelligible information they can make sense of. Think back to the days before you were a student. Would you understand words like bronchoscopy, biopsy, oncology and prognosis? In our quest for providing information there is a danger that we give too much. Look at the amount of information that is available as leaflets, booklets, videos and tapes and via countless Internet sites. Some are excellent, but some are poorly constructed and presented. If you choose to give written information read it carefully first so that you know the contents. If you are working on a ward where you feel the written information could be improved, bring it to the attention of the senior staff. Healthcare staff often criticise patients for using information found on the Internet. The so-called 'expert patient' is becoming more common and it is our responsibility to discuss such information with the patient so that myth can be separated from reality. A qualified colleague may be able to give an honest appraisal of its value.

Handling the difficult conversation – a systematic approach

- Seek further information – use reflective questioning techniques
- Allow the person to tell you their story
- Clarify your understanding of the information
- Decide on your response:
    - Offer the person a choice – honest full information, or limited information. Do they want someone with them?
    - Refer on to someone senior
- Give small amounts of information, then stop
- Invite questions
- Repeat the preceding two bullet points as much as is necessary
- Finally – summarise the conversation – tell the person what happens next

As a final check it is common to ask, 'Do you understand?'. Most patients will say 'Yes'. Instead, try saying something like, 'We have talked about a lot of things, can I just check I have explained clearly. Please can you tell me what you understand from what I have said?'. You may be surprised to hear that your clear message has not been received and understood, but you have an opportunity to explain again.

We should expect patients to retain only a small proportion of what we tell them, so it is essential to go back later that day or soon after. It is likely that they may have thought of some questions to ask you.

You will notice that the emphasis in this strategy is on offering choice, giving small amounts of information only and constantly cross-checking understanding. Remember our discussion on the unreliability of perception at the beginning of this chapter. The sequence offered here relates directly to that.

 Reflective activity

Case study: Steven

Steven was admitted to a surgical ward after having had investigations for a hoarse voice. The next day he was to have a laryngectomy and would be nursed in intensive care for a few days. On the day before Steven's surgery we went to see Steven with a student nurse to complete a pre-operative visit.

We greeted Steven, introduced ourselves and I explained the purpose of our visit: to tell Steven what would happen to him when he came to the Intensive Care Unit.

'Can I stop you there son?', Steven said with a hint of anger in his voice and in his eyes. 'I have been seen by the house officer, the senior house officer, the registrar and the consultant'. I have been seen by the theatre nurse, the anaesthetic nurse and now you two. All of them have told me what they are going to do to me, how it won't hurt it will just be uncomfortable and oh, by the way, you won't be able to talk but you can just write down what you want'.

'No-one has told me how I am going to cope with all this. Oh and by the way, I can't write even though I run my own business. Most of the sentences these people used finished with – OK? All right? No it isn't okay, it's bloody terrifying. You lot just haven't a bloody clue.'

Response: Steven quite rightly felt patronised and overwhelmed not only by the amount of information he was given, but by the attitude of the staff he met, who in his opinion were more concerned with telling him facts rather than listening to him. Bear this in mind when you next go on duty.

Using reflective questioning

This technique is perhaps one of the most useful and easily remembered of all the communication skills that have been developed. It simply involves reflecting back the initial difficult question to the person in order to get more information. Doing so will give you a much more complete understanding of the nature and context of why the question has been asked and of how you can respond to it.

Let's take some of the examples used earlier and offer a reflective response to illustrate the technique.

Question	Reflective response
How long have I got?	**How** long do you think you may have?
Does this mean the cancer has come back?	**What** makes you think the cancer has come back?
What will it be like?	**What** exactly do you mean by 'it'?
Have I got cancer?	**What** makes you think you may have cancer?

 Reflective point

Notice the two key words highlighted in bold in the text are '**How**' and '**What**'. Both these words were used to frame an open and reflective question and will offer the person the opportunity for a conversational response. If you can remember nothing else, then '**How**' and '**What**' will help you considerably.

What can I say?

This is the single most asked question of any educator in palliative care. Unfortunately the master checklist of perfect responses to every possible question does not exist and probably never will. But there are some useful questions, and statements and prompts that can help you to develop a conversation.

- Would you like to talk?
- Would you like to tell me what's on your mind?
- What is it really like to be you?
- What's troubling you?
- In the time that's left, what is important to you?
- Is there anything I can say/do to help?
- How do you feel now you have had a chance to speak to the doctor?
- Have you any regrets?
- Is there anything you can do to put things right?
- What do you really enjoy?
- Tell me what it was like to be an engineer/manager/teacher?

Notice how person-centred and open these questions are. Some are factually oriented, others are more about feelings and some ask the person to review their values, life skills and achievements. Sensitive listening, attending and questioning will have enormous benefits for patients and staff.

 Reflective activity

When you have a quiet moment scan down the list of questions offered above and relate them to a major life event you have experienced that caused you distress. Pick out those you feel would have been really helpful at the time and those which you feel may have been intrusive or difficult to respond to. Practice the helpful ones when you are next on duty.

Tip: Only select two or three; you will not remember any more and if you momentarily forget them at the bedside, recall your own life event to act as a trigger.

The value of silence

Silence is when nothing happens – or is it? A lot of active and useful thinking goes on in a silence that is valuable to both the patient and the nurse.

The patient's mind will be far from empty; he will be searching for words to express complex and perhaps tragic feelings. Throughout life most of us get little opportunity to do this. We find it difficult to express our thoughts, feelings and needs when we are fit and well. When we are ill it is much more difficult. It is hard to find the right words and our thoughts become confused. When we are in this frame of mind remember that the slightest interruption can break our train of thought and set us back a long way. Just as spaces are needed on a page to emphasise the words, so pauses and silences in a conversation are necessary to emphasise what is being said (Booth, 2000).

 Reflective activity

Find a colleague in your area who you know has these skills and observe their interactions with patients and family carefully. Make notes afterwards regarding the context of the conversation and whether you felt the silence was helpful or not. Next time you encounter such a silence, practise extending it by small but significant amounts. Revisit your notes and comment on how you felt doing this and how the patient reacted.

Further developing our communication skills

This is a lifelong process. We learn our skills by watching and listening to others and by learning about how others perceive our skill levels.

- **Identify your own style**: Listen carefully to yourself and ask trusted colleagues to give you honest feedback.
- **Listen attentively to others**: Reflect carefully on their style and techniques, accept their strengths and reject their weaknesses. Note useful phrases and gestures. Don't attempt to learn a script, but adapt the style of colleagues.
- **Practice, practice, practice**: Role play with fellow students, colleagues and other willing and suitable volunteers. Ask for feedback.
- **Record your practice**: Take a video and sound recording of your role plays and review it carefully. You will almost certainly baulk at this idea initially, as few of us are comfortable seeing ourselves on film and listening to our recorded voice, but there is no better way of seeing our skills as others see them. You will be your own fiercest critic, but you need also to learn to acknowledge your skills. Self-affirmation is good and will boost your self-esteem.

Questions about euthanasia

A request for euthanasia is usually a plea for better care. Most people are not keen to die earlier than they need to, and therefore such a request merits careful exploration. The phrase 'help me to die' when explored usually means 'help me'. All such questions or statements should be taken seriously and using the techniques outlined so far in this chapter allow the patient time to talk it through. There is almost always something constructive that can be offered to help.

Reflective point

There is no right or wrong way to die and we will encounter much sadness, distress, disappointment regret and guilt in addition to the satisfaction of sometimes witnessing the mending of relationships. There will always be a small number of people who persist in their requests for medical assistance to die. This is a complex ethical debate which is explored in more detail in Chapter 5, but for the person asking the question it is **their** death and no one else's. We only die once in our lives; therefore there is no second chance to get it right for our patients. They deserve our full attention, respect and help. There will be no second chance.

Responding to distress

It is likely that we have walked past the bed of many patients unaware of the distress they are feeling. As we search for answers we soon realise that they are hard to find. Cassidy (1988, p. 64) offers something helpful, and powerful to reflect upon:

> Slowly I learn about the importance of powerlessness. I experience it in my life and I live with it in my work. The secret is not to be afraid of it – not to run away. The dying know we are not God.... All they ask is that we do not desert them.

Think carefully about this statement. Cassidy tells us that sharing a difficult question is more important than answering it if our patients are to feel cared for rather than deserted. Communicating with patients and families is not about having all the answers and fixing all the problems. First and foremost we must learn to distinguish between the fixable and the unfixable. Communicating is about sharing the journey, the darkness and the light.

Think about what it would be like if you were living with an advancing illness like cancer, MND, HIV or heart disease. If you had to describe your communication needs what would they be? They would probably include the following:

■ Information about your illness, how it will affect you and how to cope with it
■ Honesty
■ Professionals who talk to each other
■ Someone to listen to you
■ Someone to be with you but not to talk
■ Everyday conversation about what is happening in the world
■ Opportunities to say goodbye
■ Companionship
■ Love and affection

Timely and open communication is a cornerstone of palliative care. Without effective communication, pain and symptom control cannot be achieved no matter how much knowledge we have about the latest drugs.

Communication is not and never has been a simple process and one must remember that it takes place within highly complex social systems. Although we have considered some of the mechanisms and attitudes required to facilitate effective communication, it would be presumptuous to suggest that it is as simple as learning a set of skills. In addition to learning these skills, attention must be paid to the complex relationships where you work.

Responding to patients and their families

We become adept at social chat and, to some extent, giving factual information. Unfortunately, at times we sometimes enter into collusion with relatives and develop techniques which block rather than facilitate meaningful discussion. Cooley (2000) explains how to guide your conversations to ensure they are based more on facilitating than on blocking.

Blocking tactics

☹ Changing the subject
☺ Inappropriate information
☹ Selective attention (to physical but not psychological)

☹ Normalising or belittling comments
☹ Premature false reassurance
☹ Leading, closed and multiple questions
☹ Passing the buck
☹ Changing focus to the relatives
☹ Jollying along and personal chit chat

Blocking: some examples

Patient: I feel awful today, I think I'll stay in bed this morning.
Nurse: Come on now don't be a lazy bones, it's a lovely day outside.
Patient: I am finding it very difficult to sleep
Nurse: Mmm... and how's your appetite?
Patient: This is much worse than I thought it would be.
Nurse: And how is your wife coping?
Patient: This wound is very sore when I move
Nurse: Yes everybody finds that.
Patient: How do you think I am getting on nurse?
Nurse: Have you asked the doctor?

Facilitation techniques: be aware of your skills

☺ Let the patient speak
☺ Active listening
☺ Acknowledging
☺ Picking up cues
☺ Open questions
☺ Warmth and empathy
☺ Clarification
☺ Confrontation
☺ Information
☺ Repetition and reiteration
☺ Conversation encouragers, e.g. nodding, smiling, touch
☺ Paraphrasing and reflecting
☺ Talk about feelings, emotions and distress
☺ Manage silences carefully without being tempted to rush in
☺ Be tentative

Facilitating techniques: some examples

Patient: I feel awful today, I think I'll stay in bed this morning.
Nurse: That's not like you John. What do you mean when you say awful?
Patient: I am finding it very difficult to sleep
Nurse: That must be distressing, is there anything I can do to help?
Patient: This is much worse than I thought it would be.
Nurse: What is it that you feel is so bad?
Patient: This wound is very sore when I move
Nurse: Let's have a look; I am sure there is something I can do to help.
Patient: How do you think I am getting on nurse?
Nurse: There seems to be something worrying you, would you like to tell me about it?

Aim for more ☺ and less ☹!

A word about euphemisms

The English language in general and healthcare language in particular is full of euphemisms. Death, dying and cancer have their own language which can seriously hamper effective communication.
   Examples:

- **Cancer**: Something nasty, something awful, the big one, the big C, the crab
- **Death and dying**: Gone, gone to sleep, gone to heaven, gone to be with the angels, passed away, passed on, passed over

   It is essential that we are crystal clear when we are communicating with patients and their families, as the following examples show.

Nurse: I am very sorry but Bill has just gone [meaning Bill is dead].
Bill's wife: OK nurse, I'll nip to the shops and call in when he comes back.
Patient: Nurse, how long do you think I have got? (Meaning how long before I go to theatre).
Nurse: Mmm, err, well it's too soon to say I think we will have to wait until you come back.

The issue of collusion

Many nurses in the course of their daily work have come across the issue of relatives, doctors or indeed fellow nurses colluding to deny the patient information that they are entitled to know. In a palliative care context this can be particularly difficult, because the information being hidden frequently concerns the diagnosis of a major life-shortening condition. It is important therefore to clarify what good practice is in this area and to offer some practical advice regarding handling such situations. The first question to ask is why do health professionals and families engage with collusion in the first place, when quite clearly the patients' rights are potentially being compromised.

The rationale for such actions is really quite simple; we feel that we will do the person harm if they are told the truth, we don't have the skills to give the information, or that we are not allowed to tell the truth. The reality more often for health professionals is that denying the patient information is an easy option in the short term and saves time when we are busy.

 Reflective point

There is no evidence that giving the person information, where requested, related to their diagnosis or prognosis will cause them harm. If this excuse is used by any practitioner as a reason to deny the person information it *must* be challenged. Perhaps the most pertinent response to such a request is:

Show me the evidence to support your position?

I can guarantee they will not be able to.

The Nursing and Midwifery Council's 2008 Code of Conduct (NMC, 2008) is not as explicit in its wording regarding this element of care as the 2004 version, but the role of the nurse as an advocate for our patient and the responsibility to provide information so that informed choices can be made is enshrined in this one simple phrase within the code:

You must act as an advocate for those in your care, helping them to access relevant health and social care, information and support (NMC, 2008)

Alongside this guidance are clear and unequivocal statements about good communication and the need to avoid collusion within recent government strategy documents on cancer and palliative care (NICE, 2004; DoH, 2008).

3.3 Good communication is a prerequisite for enabling patients and carers to make informed decisions about care. Communication in which patients are encouraged to participate and to direct the flow of the communication is likely to result in improved patient outcomes. It can bring not only greater understanding, but also a heightened ability to participate in the decision-making process, better health-related quality of life and a better experience of care (NICE, 2004. p. 60)

Notice the emphasis on partnership, choice and being person-centred; all elements that conform to good practice in both nursing and all other allied health professions. Perhaps the most significant statements regarding honesty and avoiding collusion are the following ones (NICE, 2004, p. 61):

3.9 Any significant news, such as a diagnosis, should be communicated honestly to a patient with the minimum of delay.

3.10 The outcome of significant consultations should be recorded in the patient's notes, with the patient being offered a permanent record of important points. Patients should be offered the opportunity to review discussions at key consultations at a later date.

You will notice from these two statements that they do not specify who it is that is giving the information and recording it. This is deliberate, because it is now widely recognised that many clinical nurses are actively involved in the giving of such information and it is seen as a key part of their role.

 Reflective point

Whilst it is the primary responsibility of medical practitioners to deliver news of diagnosis, prognosis and treatment options, responsibility also extends to the nurses directly involved in caring for the patient to support, clarify and explain such information – frequently after the doctor has gone. Nurses are likely to be the first health professional at the bedside of the patient immediately after such consultations and cannot abrogate responsibility for this role in the mistaken belief that it is not part of their job.

The consequences of collusion for the patient are simple: they carry on their life in blissful ignorance and freedom from emotional pain with less stress, and the inevitability of knowing is 'put off'. If this is the patient's choice then this should be respected. Just because we may know the information and have a desire to give it does not make it correct that we should (Vivian, 2006). Good practice dictates that there are several key questions that health professionals need to ask themselves:

- What does the patient know already?
- Does the patient want to know any more information?
- Does the patient need to know?
- Has the patient been given these choices?
- Would they like someone from their family to be with them?
- Have they worked it out already?

The consequences for the family who engage in collusion are equally simple: the difficult task of telling their loved one is 'put off' and this is justified by a feeling that they are helping and protecting. Unfortunately, such actions often build a web of deceit, conspiracy and lies that is hard to sustain.

There is the belief that hope will be destroyed if the truth is known, but hope is based on knowledge and dreams, not on ignorance. Collusion in the family is almost always an act of love and arises from a need to protect the person from the painful reality. As such, those who collude are convinced they are acting in the patient's best interest (Costello, 2000).

In legal and ethical terms the patient always has primacy. A mentally competent patient has the right to determine who shall be informed about his or her medical condition. All rights of friends or family are subsidiary to this. If a patient decides not to share information, although that may be perceived to be an aggressive or vengeful action it cannot be countermanded by the professional at the family's request. Similarly, however, well intentioned, a relative stating that 'the patient is not to be told under any circumstances' they do not have primacy over the explicit wishes of the patient if they want full disclosure (Beauchamp and Childress, 2008).

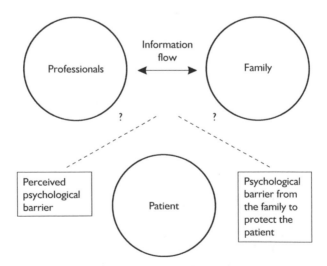

Figure 7.1 The circle of collusion which denies the patient information (Becker, 1999).

The family's feelings should not be ignored and have validity. They are closest to the person and know them best, which is double edged, because although they can anticipate to a certain degree how the person may react, they are also emotionally involved and therefore not in the best position to make a balanced judgement. The feelings and opinions of family and friends, therefore, although secondary to those of the patient, must be acknowledged even if their wishes or instructions cannot be followed.

 ## Reflective activity

Some staff in clinical areas insist on citing what they believe is hospital/unit policy not to tell patients important information when they request it. What is the policy in your area and does it provide explicit guidance based on best evidence?

NB: If challenged to become complicit in a collusion situation, the most appropriate response is to request the evidence that supports such an action. In effect there is none, so very rarely is such a stance sustainable. You are not obliged to go along with custom and practice if you believe that practice is against the patients' best interest. In reality, however, if you are at all unsure you must err on the side of caution in the first instance. It's okay to say to the patient 'I don't know, but I will find someone who does'.

How do we respond to a collusion request?

With fellow health and professionals and families alike the responses given should follow a similar stance. Firstly, using an open reflective questioning technique as discussed earlier in this chapter, explore

- What the patient knows already
- Do they want to know any more information?
- Have they been given the choice?
- Do they want all the information or just a little?
- Would they like someone from their family to be with them?
- Finally – have they worked it out already and are just needing confirmation?

When you have done that you will be in a position to make a decision whether to inform the patient or not. If you choose to do so be sure that the content and context of the conversation is reported immediately afterwards to the person in charge and a written record is made of this. There are no guarantees as to the outcome of this conversation, but you are accountable for your actions, both as a student to more senior staff and when qualified to the NMC and your employer.

Remember: no other health professional or family member can ask you to lie to the patient – that would directly contravene the NMC Code of Conduct (2008). Medical staff cannot be expected to be aware of a nurse's professional duty and it is appropriate and correct to state our position. Equally, family members have no knowledge of such matters – all they want is to protect their loved one, but do understand that if we are asked a direct question by the patient we cannot lie.

This simple quotation taken from the book *The Death of Ivan Ilyich* by Leo Tolstoy (1960) sums up the futility and damage that collusion can cause.

> What tormented Ivan Ilyich the most was the pretence, which for some reason they all kept up, that he was merely ill and not dying and that he need only stay quiet and carry out the doctor's orders and that some great change for the better would result.
>
> But he knew nothing would come of it except still more agonising, suffering and death. The pretence made him wretched: it tormented him that they refused to admit what they knew and he knew to be a fact but persisted in lying to him and forced him to be a party to that lie. Deceit, this deceit enacted over him up to the very eve of his death: this lying which could only degrade the awful solemn act of his death was horribly painful to Ivan Ilyich.
>
> This falsity around and within him did more than anything to poison Ivan Illyich's last days.

Conclusion

This chapter has not concerned itself with the promotion or explanation of a number of widely accepted and highly successful frameworks with which to tackle difficult questions. That is not say that we cannot learn from them. Each has their merits, but most are specifically designed for medical staff usage, are reliant on a one-to-one scenario in a private situation and can be difficult to remember in the bustle of a busy clinical environment. The techniques offered here are an eclectic mix, taken and adapted from some of these frameworks and sprinkled with a modicum of learnt experience over many years in clinical practice. If you would like to learn more about these frameworks to further develop your skills, the list offered below will point you in the right direction

- Buckman (1992)   6 step protocol
- Kaye (1996)   10 step protocol
- Faulkner (1998)   6 step protocol
- Baile *et al.* (2000)   SPIKES framework

Palliative care is based on the firm foundation of sensitive open communication between patients, families and professionals. The good news is that we are slowly but surely becoming better at it as confidence grows and skills rise. The bad news is that in our well-developed healthcare system there are still far too many instances of poor communication being reported through complaints systems. I firmly believe that the will is there from the majority of health professionals to get it right and we need to acknowledge the countless excellent instances of good practice that happen daily that are quickly forgotten and go unreported. If a tally were kept of these examples I am certain it would more than counterbalance the negative reports by a very large statistical margin.

The future is very much in our own hands. Pre-registration curricula for nursing, medicine and all allied professions have been adapted and improved over the last decade to reflect a higher emphasis on good communication skills. Postgraduate opportunities abound, both through the auspices of local hospice training departments and modular schemes at universities. The Advanced Communication Skills programme (Connected, 2009) is a major government-funded initiative that for the first time is attempting to push forward an accredited and standardised course for senior health professionals engaged in direct and sensitive communication at the end of life. It has only come about as a result of intense lobbying by palliative and cancer care clinicians over the last two decades and with significant government backing has the potential to reach out across the UK, targeting key staff to equip them with the requisite knowledge, confidence and core skills to influence communication where it really matters – at the bedside of the patient.

Job satisfaction can be hard to achieve in our complex and hard pressed healthcare system that is continually under the media spotlight. It is easy to succumb to the pressures of such demands and lose sight of what really matters. Good communication skills in a palliative care context role modelled well in clinical practice can provide us with some of the most powerful learning experiences of our career. Such skills are not the preserve of the specialist and are accessible to all nurses. Just remember that it is the small things that really matter most – if you get those right then the rest will be so much easier, as our concluding quote so aptly demonstrates:

> Too often we underestimate the power of a touch, a smile, a kind word, a listening ear, an honest compliment, or the smallest act of caring, all of which have the potential to turn a life around (Leo Busgalia, 1925–1998; US author and lecturer)

References

Baile, W., Buckman, R., Lenzi, R., Glober, G., Beale, E. A. Kudelka, A. P. (2000) SPIKES – a 6 step protocol for delivering bad news: application to the patient with cancer. *The Oncologist*, **5**, 302–11.

Beauchamp, T. L. and Childress, J. F. (2008) *Principles of Biomedical Ethics*, 6th edn. Oxford University Press, New York.

Becker, R. (1999) Teaching communication skills with the dying across cultural boundaries. *British Journal of Nursing*, **8**(15), 938–42.

Booth, R. (2000) Spirituality: sharing the journey. In: *Stepping into Palliative Care. A Handbook for Community Professionals* (ed. J. Cooper). Radcliffe Medical Press, Oxford.

Buckman, R. (1992) *How to Break Bad News: A Guide for Health Care Professionals*. Papermac, Basingstoke.

Buckman, R. (2005) Communication in palliative care: a practical guide. In: *Death, Dying and Bereavement* (eds. D. Dickenson, M. Johnson and J. S. Katz). Open University Press, London, in association with Sage Publications.

Busaglia, L. (2009) http://www.quotationspage.com/quote/30921.html. Accessed: 9 September 2009.

Cassidy, S. (1988) *Sharing the Darkness: the Spirituality of Caring*. Darton, Longman & Todd, London.

Connected (2009) http://www.connected.nhs.uk/. Accessed: 29 June 2009.

Cooley, C. (2000) Communication skills in palliative care. *Professional Nurse*, **15**(9), 6603–5.

Costello, J. (2000) Truth telling and the dying patient: a conspiracy of silence? *International Journal of Palliative Nursing*, **6**(8), 398–405.

Covey, S. (1989) *The Seven Habits of Highly Effective People*. Simon & Schuster, London.

Department of Health (2005) *The Mental Capacity Act*. Retrieved September 2009 from http://www.dh.gov.uk/publications/.

Department of Health (2008) *End of Life Care Strategy. Promoting High Quality Care for All Adults at the End of Life*. DoH, London.

Dunlop, R. (1999) *The Times*, 10 June 1999, p. 21.

Faulkner, A. (1998) *When the News is Bad: a Guide for Health Professionals*. Stanley Thornes, Cheltenham.

Jones, A. (1999) A heavy and blessed experience: a psychoanalytical study of community Macmillan nurses and their role in serious illness and palliative care. *Journal of Advanced Nursing*, **30**(6), 1297–303.

Kaye, P. (1996) *Breaking Bad News: a 10 Step Approach*. EPL, Northampton.

National Institute for Clinical Excellence (2004) *Improving Supportive and Palliative Care for Adults with Cancer: The Manual*. NICE, London.

Nursing and Midwifery Council (2008) *Standards of Conduct, Performance and Ethics for Nurses and Midwives*. NMC, London.

Rowling, J.K. (1997) *Harry Potter and The Philosopher's Stone*. Bloomsbury, London.

Randall, F. and Downie, R. S. (1999) *Palliative Care Ethics*, 2nd edn. Oxford University Press, Oxford.

Smith, R. C. (2001) *Patient-Centred Interviewing: an Evidence-Based Method*, 2nd edn. Lippincott, Williams & Wilkins, Philadelphia.

Tolstoy, L. (1960) *The Death of Ivan Ilyich*. Penguin Books, London.

Vivian, R. (2006) Truth telling in palliative care nursing: the dilemmas of collusion. *International Journal of Palliative Nursing*, **12**(7), 341–9.

Useful websites

EPERC
http://www.mywhatever.com/cifwriter/library/eperc/fastfact/ff06.html

Breaking Bad News
http://www.breakingbadnews.co.uk/index.asp

University College Medical School
http://www.pcps.ucl.ac.uk/commskills/student_handbook/bad_news.htm

Auckland District Health Board
http://www.adhb.govt.nz/downloads/res_conf/breaking-bad-news-talk.ppt

Skills Cascade.com
http://www.skillscascade.com/badnews.htm#Preparation:

American Family Physician Journal
http://www.aafp.org/afp/20011215/1975.html

Ethics in Medicine
http://depts.washington.edu/bioethx/topics/badnws.html

Phuket Gazette
http.//www.pcps.ucl.ac.uk/commskills/student_handbook/bad_news.htm

☑ Chapter links to the Nursing and Midwifery Council Standards of Conduct, Performance and Ethics for Nurses and Midwives (2008)

Section I: Make the care of people your first concern, treating them as individuals and respecting their dignity

Treat people as individuals
- You must treat people as individuals and respect their dignity
- You must treat people kindly and considerately

- You must act as an advocate for those in your care, helping them to access relevant health and social care, information and support

Collaborate with those in your care
- You must listen to the people in your care and respond to their concerns and preferences
- You must make arrangements to meet people's language and communication needs
- You must share with people, in a way they can understand, the information they want or need to know about their health

Section 2: Work with others to protect and promote the health and wellbeing of those in your care, their families and carers, and the wider community

Share information with your colleagues
- You must keep your colleagues informed when you are sharing the care of others

Work effectively as part of a team
- You must work cooperatively within teams and respect the skills, expertise and contributions of your colleagues
- You must be willing to share your skills and experience for the benefit of your colleagues
- You must consult and take advice from colleagues when appropriate
- You must make a referral to another practitioner when it is in the best interests of someone in your care

Section 3: Provide a high standard of practice and care at all times

Keep clear and accurate records
- You must keep clear and accurate records of the discussions you have, the assessments you make, the treatment and medicines you give and how effective these have been
- You must complete records as soon as possible after an event has occurred
- You must not tamper with original records in any way
- You must ensure any entries you make in someone's paper records are clearly and legibly signed, dated and timed
- You must ensure any entries you make in someone's electronic records are clearly attributable to you
- You must ensure all records are kept confidentially and securely

☑ Self-assessment test

1. When fielding difficult questions from a patient after they have been told of their life limiting diagnosis it is good practice to:
   A   Divert their attention to other matters so that they don't get upset
   B   Seek out someone else more senior to handle the conversation
   C   Ask the person to tell you about their understanding of the issues now facing them
   D   Offer encouraging phrase that it will be okay

2. Self-perception of visual, auditory and written communication is:
   A   Always reliable
   B   Generally reliable
   C   Part of professional practice
   D   Open to interpretation

3. When using reflective questioning there are certain key words that can help you frame your response. They include:
   A   How, why
   B   What, how
   C   Pardon, have
   D   Could, what

4. Which of the following statements is correct?
   A   Hope can be better maintained by only giving the patient selective information
   B   The family ultimately have the final say over whether the patient is told of their diagnosis, because they know them best
   C   Requests by any health professional to engage in collusion to deny a competent person information – even though well intentioned, should always be challenged
   D   Only doctors have the right to give difficult information to patients

5. Good listening skills are:
   A   A natural and intuitive ability that cannot really be taught
   B   A simple and passive process which is all about paying attention
   C   All about personality, charm and common sense
   D   Hard work and demand close attention to both verbal and non-verbal elements and plenty of practice

CHAPTER 8

The nature of pain and suffering

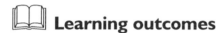 *My name is Graham, I have advanced cancer. At first there was no pain now it hurts everywhere. They give me lots of medicines but don't seem to understand how much death and leaving loved ones hurts. Very soon I will be a pile of ashes. Please try to understand, this is what hurts most.*

📖 Learning outcomes

After reading this chapter and completing the reflective activities the learner will be able to:

- Define pain and suffering in a palliative care context
- Describe the causes of pain and relate these to nursing practice
- Understand the principles that underpin the concept of total pain

Introduction

Understanding the nature of pain and suffering is a complex challenge for nurses in any environment, but is essential knowledge before the accurate assessment and management of that pain is attempted. The human body is far more than just a biophysical entity and all its component parts interact and affect each other when serious illness and chronic pain strike. It is possible, for example to suffer extreme psychological and spiritual distress and yet have no physical signs of pain as we would understand it. It is also possible to observe someone in severe physical pain who may choose to ignore it or even consider that it is a necessary part of their suffering. The experience of pain therefore is totally unique to the individual and by its very nature is entirely subjective. It is this that makes dealing with pain such an immense challenge for nurses and also one of the most rewarding aspects of palliative care.

This chapter will look closely at the way pain is described and defined and what we understand are the most common causes of pain. It will conclude by examining the concept of 'total pain' as first termed by Dame Cicely Saunders in 1967 and how this fits with today's complex caring environments. There are a selection of stimulating and thought-provoking activities interspersed throughout the chapter that are designed to help you reflect on your knowledge of pain and your approach to patients when they ask for your help.

Whilst the prescription of appropriate medication to relieve physical pain is the direct responsibility of doctors it is the nurse and their unique relationship with the patient who is in the best position to see the complete picture as presented by the patient and to bring about change to alleviate pain and suffering whatever its nature.

What is meant by 'pain and suffering'

Of all the problems that people with advanced illness have to face pain is often the one that is feared the most. Accordingly, freedom from pain is one of the fundamental aims of care for any patient. You may already have thought quite a lot about pain and indeed have encountered many patients in your work suffering from both acute and chronic pain. There are many definitions that exist in the literature, so it is prudent that we take a look at some of these to see just how they fit with the lived experience of the patient.

1. 'An unpleasant sensory and emotional experience associated with actual or potential tissue damage, or described in terms of such damage' (IASP, 1986)
2. 'A category of complex experiences not a single sensation produced by a single stimulus' (Melzack and Wall, 1991)
3. 'Pain is what the experiencing person says it is, existing whenever he says it does' (McCaffery, 1983).

Each of these definitions is accurate and they all express rather different aspects of pain. Take a look again and ask yourself which of these definitions you are most drawn to. It will most likely be the final one, from Margo McCaffery. The emphasis in this definition lies in the subjectivity of pain. That is, it points clearly to the fact that pain is something which can only be felt, described and measured by the person experiencing it. Definitions 1 and 2 each describe specific physiological aspects of pain but take no account of its subjectivity.

If you are to accept this subjectivity then it implies that you must suspend any judgement; not an easy thing to do in many over-stretched and understaffed clinical areas. One of the most common concerns expressed by patients is that they feel some nurses and doctors disbelieve them when they report pain. Through her definition McCaffery is communicating the view that if you are really to help someone in pain you must first ask the patient about that pain and accept what they are telling you.

 ## Reflective activity

Pain is a very common experience for all of us. Think back over the last six months or so and make a note of any pain you have experienced.

Feedback: Your list may contain some of the following:

- Headache
- Back pain
- Toothache
- Menstrual pain
- Arthritic pain
- Indigestion

You may have included pain that has a more psychological origin such as the pain of losing a loved one through death, divorce or separation, or the pain of a broken relationship or even being made redundant from your job. From this simple exercise we can learn two important lessons.

In everyday life some degree of pain is common. Patients with advancing illnesses frequently experience pain that is *not* due to their disease. Pain is not simply a physical phenomenon. Psychological, social, intellectual and spiritual issues affect the way we experience pain. Neglecting any of the contributing factors will result in poor pain management.

Definitions of suffering

It is difficult to reduce suffering to a simple definition and most authors agree that the personal, subjective experience of suffering will always defy full analysis (Becker, 2009). Suffering is described as essentially a negative experience involving distress, discomfort, and endurance. Even when pain is well controlled, patients can suffer. In life we hope for many things, but at the core is the desire to find peace, love and understanding, wholeness and meaning. Knowing that one is dying, saying goodbye to loved ones and friends, losing the ability to walk, enjoy food, make love... all contribute to suffering. Yet the extremes of human deprivation and the experience of terminal illness teach us that, even in the worst circumstances, peace is possible (Mount 2003).

Staff who care for the dying may suffer too. Students sometimes feel this more acutely than qualified colleagues who have developed a social structure and shared coping mechanisms. Students can feel a sense of failure, 'I didn't know what to say' or 'I didn't know what to do'. They experience anger, guilt and loss of control. They don't feel involved in decision-making supervision or post-death review meetings.

Those who constantly work with dying patients are exposed to serious illness, disability, loss, pain and death. They stare suffering in the face on a daily basis and if suffering is not acknowledged this can lead to exhaustion, stress and damaged relationships.

Surprisingly quality of life and a sense of being healthy do not correlate with a sense of wellbeing. It is possible to experience profound physical disability and, at the same time, a high quality of life. Viktor Frankl's book, *Man's Search for Meaning* (Frankl, 1959) tells of his experiences while captive in a Nazi concentration camp during the Second World War. He concluded that our human quest is not for fame and fortune but for meaning. Meaning, he suggests may be found in five domains:

- Things created or accomplished
- Things left to others, to be remembered by
- Things we believe in
- Things loved
- The experience of suffering.

When hope of cure is no longer realistic the above five domains serve as prompts for our conversations with the dying and bereaved.

 Reflective activity

Below are a number of questions which can be asked. Take some time out now and ask *yourself* these very questions and keep a note of your responses.

- When you look back over your life, what are you most proud of?
- What do you feel you will be remembered for?
- Who and what have you loved?
- What experiences have you in your life that have had a profound effect on you?

Feedback: I expect you found that quite difficult to do. For our patients these are important questions and can help them gain a context and sense of meaning for their whole life and not just the period of pain and suffering that is most prominent at that time. For ourselves it can give an invaluable insight into the values we hold and the way we lead our own lives.

The relief of pain and suffering is clearly spelt out in the internationally accepted WHO definition of palliative care (WHO, 2004), so it is therefore widely accepted as a prime imperative of good palliative care wherever it takes place. It places an onus on us to think holistically about the patient and the totality of their situation.

The uniqueness of pain

You may have noticed that when patients talk about their pain they use very different language and gestures to describe that pain and for many it is a difficult experience to find the right words for. This is because it is such an intense and subjective experience that it draws on and saps our reserves of energy and ability to express ourselves.

 ## Reflective activity

Spend a minute or two thinking about the most recent pain experience you have had then write down words or phrases that come into your mind that would help someone else understand your pain. When you have done this find another person (a friend or colleague) and ask them to do the same exercise. Compare what you have both written down and look for common words or phrases. Also try to share some of the emotions, fears and worries you had and the way it made you feel.

Feedback: You may well have found that even if you chose a similar pain experience your words were quite different to the other person. This is because the person's perception of that pain is wholly unique to them. The differences are illuminating, but I am sure you will have also found some similarities.

For example, bone pain is often described as a dull nagging ache that is constant, whereas nerve pain, by contrast, is characteristically sharp in nature and can be traced along the line of the nerve itself. Traumatic tissue damage can involve skin, muscle and bone pain in what for the patient is an overwhelming mixture of different pains.

The experience of pain

It is important to contrast the differences between acute and chronic pain and look at the nature of pain tolerance and thresholds. It is generally accepted that pain that is acute in origin and nature is different from pain that is chronic. The experience of acute pain is usually of a pain short in duration as opposed to the much longer duration of chronic pain, and approaches to treating each are very different.

Definitions

- **Acute pain**: This is an event which is essentially protective and warning in nature and sends messages to the brain which say 'back off and move away'. All of us have suffered acute pain in some way, for example a burn on the hand or a kick on the shin. And we can relate to such pain much more easily than any other kind. It is generally intense but short in duration, and tends to diminish.
- **Chronic pain**: It is impossible to predict the outcome of chronic pain as it seems to serve no warning or protective function to the body. It is generally persistent and becomes progressively worse unless the cause is identified and addressed. It creates a feeling of hopelessness and frequently dominates patients' lives. It may even affect their will to live.
- **Pain threshold**: This term is used to describe the amount of noxious stimuli (for example, heat to the skin) that will cause an individual to feel pain.
- **Pain tolerance**: This refers to the amount of pain that a person can put up with. This varies depending on the presence or absence of certain factors. Hunger, tiredness and anxiety can lower a person's pain tolerance, making pain less easy to bear, whereas a good meal, rest or an interesting activity (distraction) can increase pain tolerance.

Reflective activity

Have a look at the five mini-case studies below and see which ones are either acute or chronic pain and which display a high or low tolerance within their threshold.

1. Mrs Jones, a lady in her early sixties, suffers from continual severe backache which restricts her mobility and independence. She finds it difficult to go far from her house and even simple household jobs are increasingly difficult for her. Since the cause of her pain is unknown and all the treatments she has tried are ineffective she is caught in a circle of pain and depression.
2. Tim is a 16-year-old footballer who frequently gets knocks on his shin during the excitement of a football match and has large bruises which he often doesn't even notice.
3. Susan is Tim's sister who is a rather tense and anxious young lady who has few friends and complains a lot when her finger is pricked for a blood sample.

4. Harry is a soldier who had a large piece of his arm blown away by shrapnel in the heat of battle. He managed, however, to go to the aid of his fallen comrade and to drag him away from the danger zone and felt no pain from his injury for some time.

5. Mrs Smith suffers from breast cancer and has done so for nearly seven years. She has received a lot of treatment for secondaries in her bones, which give her constant pain, but she always has a smile on her face in public and spends much of her time walking the hills and swimming to raise money for her favourite cancer charity.

Feedback: Each case is very different and illustrates the complexity of the pain experience. Suggested responses may include:

1. Mrs Jones: Her back pain is clearly chronic in nature and her tolerance of it is diminishing rapidly, as evidenced by her low mood. She has also probably developed quite a high pain threshold out of the sheer necessity to get on with life.

2. Tim: His pain a very acute in nature and his immediate tolerance is quite high due to the adrenaline in his body when playing football. It's probably not until several hours after that he may experience pain associated with this injury.

3. Susan: Her pain is very acute in nature and because of her anxious personality and the anticipation of expecting pain her tolerance and pain threshold can be said to be quite low.

4. Harry: His situation is a clear indicator of battlefield pain that is life-threatening in itself, but the body's physiology in a survival crisis of high adrenaline and endorphin release in the body enables an individual to temporarily shut off the pain experience. Only much later, when the body is no longer in shock, will he feel the massive acute pain of such a severe injury.

5. Mrs Smith: This is a classic example of an individual suffering chronic debilitating long-term pain that is both nociceptive and neuropathic (see below) in origin. Her psychological attitude to her pain and coping strategies have been used very effectively. In reality, her pain threshold may be quite low, but she has learned to increase her pain tolerance by using distraction activities that are focused on other things, such as walking and swimming.

Types of pain

Pain is primarily divided into two main types, nociceptive and neuropathic.

- **Nociceptive pain**: All over the body there are sensory organs in the tips of nerves which detect pain. They are called nociceptors. They transmit nerve impulses via the spinal cord to the brain. The frequency and intensity of these impulses tell us where the pain is and how severe it is. When stimulated they evoke a reflex action, such as when we touch something hot. This pain can have a physiological origin and manifest itself in conditions such as migraine, cramp or colic. It can also be the result of a disease process or trauma, such as cancer, arthritis, or infection.

■ **Neuropathic pain**: This arises when nerves which carry messages of sensation, including pain, light, touch, vibration, warmth and coldness, are compressed or damaged by disease or an accident. The pain is then felt in the area of the body supplied by that nerve. An example of this is when the herpes zoster virus becomes active, as in shingles. Severe pain is felt in blisters arising in the nerve's territory and the pain can persist long after the skin has healed.

 Reflective activity

Read the short case study below and list the kinds of pain you think that Joe is experiencing.

Case study: Joe

Joe is a 44-year-old man with advanced bowel cancer. He is admitted to hospital and during his initial discussion with the nurse she finds out the following information.

He is complaining of intense and deep-seated lower abdominal pain which is constant and wearing him out and the paracetamol he is currently taking has no effect. He also says he has pain in his shoulder. When questioned he says it comes from damage to a joint – the result of a motorcycle accident many years ago. While in the bathroom with Sam, a student nurse, Joe says 'I have a terrible pain down my right leg as well, which seems to come from nowhere like an electric shock. I am terrified waiting for it to come back and I can't sleep'.

Feedback: It is clear that Joe's lower abdominal pain is directly linked with his bowel cancer and it is therefore nociceptive pain. His shoulder pain is likely to be associated with damage to his joints, may be arthritic in origin and is clearly a nociceptive pain. The pain in his right leg, however, is almost certainly nerve related and is therefore neuropathic in origin.

Mechanisms of pain

Figure 8.1 shows a cross-section through the skin and the various receptors found there, including receptors for sensing temperature and pressure. It also

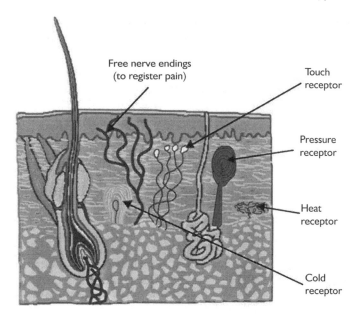

Figure 8.1 Receptors in the skin.

shows 'free nerve endings'. Stimulation of these free nerve endings, which are called nocioceptors, causes the sensation of pain.

Figure 8.2 shows a simple reflex action to a painful stimulus.

1. Sticking a pin into your finger stimulates nociceptors.

2–4. This causes a signal to be transmitted to the spinal cord. The nerve fibres are referred to as afferent, i.e. they are travelling away from the stimulus towards the central nervous system (CNS).

4–6. When the signal arrives in the spinal cord two things happen. (1) the signal is passed to a neurone in the spinal cord that transmits it up to the brain, and (2) the spinal cord itself simultaneously causes a response via efferent neurones travelling back towards the arm and hand without the need for processing by the brain. This phenomenon – not requiring the brain to process a stimulus before a response is achieved – is called a simple spinal reflex arc.

7–8. The spinal response is to send a signal through to a motor neurone (the efferent neurone), which automatically results in muscles contracting, thereby withdrawing the finger from the painful stimulus (in this case the pin).

Now that you understand a simple reflex response and why it causes pain we will turn our attention to the differences between acute and chronic pain transmission.

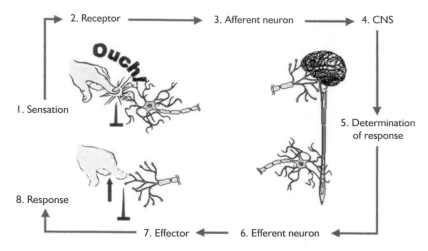

Figure 8.2 A simple reflex action to a painful stimulus.

Table 8.1 shows the differences between the fibres responsible for acute and chronic pain transmission. In particular it draws attention to the important fact that Ao fibres are myelinated (a sheath that covers some axons). This ensures a more rapid transmission than their C fibre counterparts which are unmyelinated and therefore exhibit slower transmission.

In visual terms this is better demonstrated by Figures 8.3 and 8.4.

Figure 8.3 is a schematic diagram illustrating the interplay between the peripheral and the central nervous system. Afferent neurones (part of the peripheral nervous system) all, at some point, enter the spinal cord via the dorsal route nerves then pass up the spinal cord into the brain via ascending pathways. (Although descending pathways do exist these have not been shown for the purposes of simplicity.)

Figure 8.4 shows the transmission of acute pain via the Ao fibres. The Ao fibres enter the dorsal root ganglion and synapse before ascending to the brain.

Chronic pain in contrast is transmitted via C fibres that have an additional synapse (interneurone) before ascending to the brain (Figure 8.5). The interneurone can be significant in modulating pain. This can result in various

Table 8.1 Differences between acute (Ao fibres) and chronic (C fibres) pain (Weatherall, 1996).

Ao fibres	C fibres
Early sharp pain	Later dull pain
Myelinated	Unmyelinated
Rapid transmission	Slower transmission
$4–30 \text{ m s}^{-1}$	$0.5–2 \text{ m s}^{-1}$

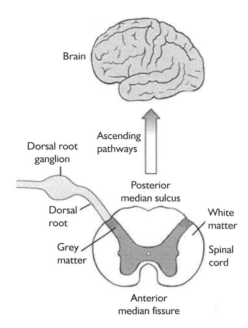

Figure 8.3 The interplay between the peripheral and the central nervous system (reproduced with kind permission from Actiq Slide Toolkit by Cephalon).

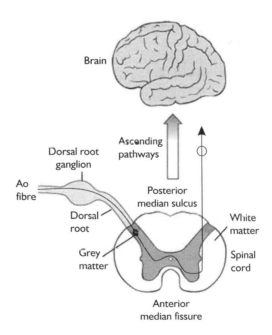

Figure 8.4 The transmission of acute pain via the Ao fibres (reproduced with kind permission from Actiq Slide Toolkit by Cephalon).

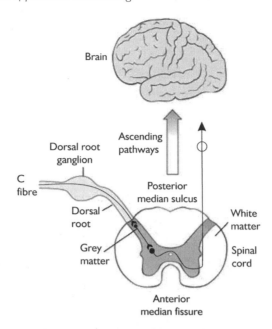

Figure 8.5 The transmission of chronic pain via the C fibres (reproduced with kind permission from Actiq Slide Toolkit by Cephalon).

sensations being experienced by the patient, it can also make the treatment of chronic pain more difficult.

Total pain

This simple and easily understood concept was first described by Cicely Saunders (1967) and brings together the idea that when viewing the patient in pain we need to consider the whole person and not just the physiological element. Total pain promotes the integration of the spiritual and the psychosocial elements as equal partners alongside the physiological to aid our understanding of the pain experience and to provide the basis of a framework for the assessment and management of pain.

The reality of pain perception

The diagram of total pain (Figure 8.6) shows a wide range of contributing factors to how we perceive pain. A key point to remember is that medication

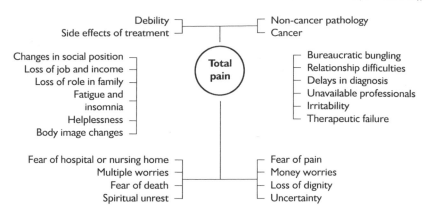

Figure 8.6 The concept of 'total pain', first described by Saunders (1967).

can influence very few of these factors. Most, if not all, can be influenced by skilled nursing. You will notice also that most of the factors cited overlap, so looking at any one in isolation is not really going to help a great deal.

To illustrate the necessity of this concept, read the conversation below.

Patient: The cancer is so painful at times but what hurt even more was that *nobody* seemed to care.

Nurse: What made you think that nobody cared?

Patient: They were all always so busy.... They gave me lots of medicine which took some of the pain away but made me very sleepy and sick. Surely they must have other things that can help you today rather than pills and potions? But you know they didn't come back to see how I was. It was as if they didn't want to be with me.

Nurse: How did that make you feel?

Patient: You can't possibly imagine anything worse. Dying alone in the midst of all these busy people, what's gone wrong?

Unfortunately this scenario is not uncommon in many caring environments even today, and demonstrates how difficult it is to address the holistic needs of our patients in an acute hospital scenario dominated by the medical, disease-oriented model of care. Embracing the concept of holism and total pain should be no contradiction for nurses, as the very notion of caring for the whole person is at the core of nursing philosophy. Yet, as we know, the art of caring often receives far less attention than the science within our increasingly complex healthcare systems.

As you look at the diagram of total pain you may also be aware that there are some things that are missing from it. Indeed it is not exhaustive of many factors that affect the person and was never intended to be, but it is meant to be representative of the primary issues that may crop up from a holistic view-point. By using a holistic model we can soon list a whole range of other factors that can affect the pain experience for the individual. This will depend on your culture, your values and beliefs, and whether you work in an old people's home or deliver care in an institution of some kind. Some examples include:

Physical
Movement and mobility
Position of the body
Clothing
Muscle tension/spasm
Posture
Rest and sleep
Infection
Constipation

Psychological
Attitudes to health and illness
Knowledge of the condition
Past experiences
Loss of control and autonomy
Depression
Anger

Environmental
Unfamiliar surroundings
Noise
Dampness
Sanitation
Extremes of temperature
Housing conditions
Pollutants

Social
Religious faith – challenged by serious illness
Cultural norms – related to pain acceptance and control
Diagnosis – related to information and who is given it
Employment – financial worries
Isolation

Studies have also shown that age and gender also pay a part in the pain experience (McCaffery, 1983) The pain of labour and childbirth is unique to the female gender and been described as all-pervading and highly subjective.

It may present itself as part nociceptive due to tissue damage during childbirth itself and part neuropathic as the weight of the unborn child presses on key nerves in the abdominal region. Conversely, some elderly people who have suffered a long-term physical infirmity for many years have adjusted their lives around the constant presence of some pain and learn to ignore it in daily life.

Reflective activity

Case study: Harry

Harry is a 45-year-old electrician who is well known to his family doctor. He is an over-anxious person who has been a regular attendee at the surgery for some years, always for trivial complaints. His usual approach to the doctor and practice nurse is 'I thought I had better come and tell you about it in case it might be serious'.

It never was serious until he turned up at the surgery after an episode of haematuria (blood in the urine). The urology department at the local hospital diagnosed a malignant tumour on his left kidney. This was removed surgically and he recovered well and went back to his life with the all-clear from the oncologist. Some time later he returned to the surgery, this time with a similar pain in his back that was constant. The GP thought that this was probably Harry overreacting as he had done in the past, particularly as he said he had been lifting things in his workshop. He prescribed a low dose of analgesics.

His wife called two weeks later to say that he was now having difficulty walking and had not passed urine for about eighteen hours – what should she do?

Harry was admitted to hospital and it was confirmed that his cancer had returned and that his prognosis was poor. He dealt with this news very badly and was aggressive to his wife and the family doctor, blaming them for his illness. When he returned home he retreated to his room and refused to talk to anyone – even the minister from his local church, who had supported him with his Christian faith for many years. Harry said, 'My faith has deserted me in my time of need. I am a good man and don't deserve this cancer, so why has God treated me this way'.

What facets of *physical* pain does Harry's case raise?

Feedback: Harry's medical and nursing needs centre around control of his cancer pain by the use of appropriate medication and helping him to maintain some mobility. His quality of life at home can be significantly enhanced if he has a walking aid and some equipment offered to adapt the house for him to get around easier.

What facets of *psychosocial* pain does Harry's case raise?

Feedback: Harry and his wife need regular emotional support that can be achieved by visits from either a community nurse or a specialist nurse in palliative care, if available. This will give them opportunities to discuss with a trusted person how they feel about the situation they are in and enable Harry's psychological health to be monitored. People in this situation, with the kind of personality that Harry has, can be at risk of clinical depression and if this should become so then appropriate medication can be started early. He may well need help financially and this can be looked at also.

What facets of *spiritual pain* does Harry's case raise?

Feedback: Facing terminal illness will challenge even the strongest of faiths, and Harry and his wife will need the continuing support that their faith community can offer. This element of pastoral support is integral to all the world's major religions and many others also and may help provide Harry with some of the profound answers he seeks. Conversely there may be no answers to these profound questions and the presence of a like-minded person of the same faith who stay with the questions and learn how to 'just be with' rather than 'do' can be a significant help. We must not forget that spiritual care embraces much more than formal religion, so Harry will need to feel cared for and not judged by all those around him.

Conclusion

In this chapter we have taken a comprehensive look at the whole concept of pain and suffering as understood from the patient's lived experience and what we know of the mechanisms of pain perception and physiology. Your study so far will give you a clearer understanding of the complex and subjective nature of this fascinating subject and will hopefully stimulate your thinking and cause you to reflect on your own practice wherever that may be. The next step is to look at how we can take this knowledge and apply it to the accurate assessment of pain in Chapter 7 and then the management of pain in Chapter 8.

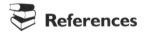 **References**

Becker, R. (2009) The teaching of hope and suffering in palliative care education: In: *Dimensions in Cancer and Palliative Care Education* (eds. L. Foyle and J. Hostad). Radcliffe Press, Oxford.

Frankl, V. E. (1959) *Man's Search for Meaning*. Beacon Press, Boston.

International Association for the Study of Pain (1986). Classification of chronic pain. Descriptions of chronic pain opioid requirements depend on previous analgesic needs syndromes and definitions of pain terms. *Pain*, S3: 1–226.

McCaffery, M. (1983) *Nursing the Patient in Pain*. Harper & Row, London.

Melzack, R. and Wall, P. D. (1991) *Textbook of Pain*. Churchill Livingstone, Edinburgh.

Mount, B. M. (2003) Existential suffering and the determinants of healing. *European Journal of Palliative Care*, **10**(2), Supplement 40–42.

Saunders, C. M. (1967) *The Management of Terminal Illness*. Hospital Medicine Publications, London.

Weatherall, D. J. (1996) *Oxford Textbook of Medicine*, 3rd edn. Oxford University Press, Oxford.

World Health Organization (2004) *WHO Definition of Palliative Care*. http://www.who.int/cancer/palliative/definition/.

Original material for this chapter was taken and adapted from the Nature of Pain online study course authored by R Becker and available at:

http://www.cancernursing.org/

Useful websites

Scottish Intercollegiate Guidelines Network – pain control
http://www.sign.ac.uk/guidelines/fulltext/44/

Pain.com
http://www.pain.com/sections/categories_of_pain/cancer/

Cancer pain.org
http://www.cancer-pain.org/

Cancer pain management in children
http://www.childcancerpain.org/

Hospice Net
http://www.hospicenet.org/html/what_is_pain.html

The Oxford Pain Internet Site
http://www.medicine.ox.ac.uk/bandolier/

🗒 Chapter links to the Nursing and Midwifery Council Standards of Conduct, Performance and Ethics for Nurses and Midwives (2008)

Section 1: Make the care of people your first concern, treating them as individuals and respecting their dignity

Treat people as individuals
- You must treat people as individuals and respect their dignity
- You must treat people kindly and considerately
- You must act as an advocate for those in your care, helping them to access relevant health and social care, information and support

Collaborate with those in your care
- You must listen to the people in your care and respond to their concerns and preferences
- You must support people in caring for themselves to improve and maintain their health
- You must recognise and respect the contribution that people make to their own care and wellbeing
- You must make arrangements to meet people's language and communication needs
- You must share with people, in a way they can understand, the information they want or need to know about their health

Section 2: Work with others to protect and promote the health and wellbeing of those in your care, their families and carers, and the wider community

Share information with your colleagues
- You must keep your colleagues informed when you are sharing the care of others

Work effectively as part of a team
- You must consult and take advice from colleagues when appropriate
- You must make a referral to another practitioner when it is in the best interests of someone in your care

Section 3: Provide a high standard of practice and care at all times

Keep your skills and knowledge up to date
- You must have the knowledge and skills for safe and effective practice when working without direct supervision
- You must take part in appropriate learning and practice activities that maintain and develop your competence and performance

☑ Self-assessment test

1. Which *one* of the following statements is correct?
   A Suffering can be measured objectively
   B A patient's suffering is a personal and subjective experience
   C Well controlled pain completely frees a patient from suffering
   D Suffering can be defined as a totally positive experience

2. Which *one* of the following statements is correct?
   A The pain threshold describes a person's level of tolerance to pain.
   B The pain threshold describes the amount of noxious stimuli that will cause an individual to feel pain.
   C The pain threshold is an objective measurement of pain.
   D The pain threshold is the same as pain tolerance.

3. Which one of the following examples describes acute pain?
   A A kick on the shin with the pain diminishing
   B A stomach ulcer with long-term pain
   C A continuous back problem with nagging pain and no relief
   D A degenerative illness leading to inability to function

4. Which one of the following is an example of neuropathic pain?
   A Migraine
   B Shingles
   C Cramp
   D Arthritis

5. What is the significance of myelinated fibres?
   A They transmit chronic pain
   B They allow for the more rapid transmission of acute pain
   C They modulate pain
   D Myelinated fibres slow transmission of pain

CHAPTER 9

The assessment of pain

 I was looking after a young man dying of motor neurone disease. He was literally helpless, and his inability to communicate meant that he shrieked louder and louder. The noise was deafening and the pain radiating from him caused distress to everyone, who were equally helpless, not knowing what to do. We needed help.

Learning outcomes

After reading this chapter and completing the reflective activities the learner will be able to:

■ Understand the principles that underpin the accurate assessment of pain in a palliative care context
■ Conduct a basic pain assessment using the tools available
■ Discuss the barriers to successful pain assessment
■ Appreciate the need for a holistic approach in the assessment of pain
■ Assess and reflect on their competency in pain assessment by use of the questionnaire offered

Introduction

The accurate assessment of pain is the cornerstone of successful pain relief and long-term management of that pain. Without it there are many facets of the patient's experience that can be missed, and consequently their pain may not be well controlled. This chapter will take a comprehensive look at all of the components of a successful holistic pain assessment and will challenge you to consider your practice in this area by the use of a case study and competencies for you to assess the level of your skills.

It is vitally important to assess the presence and severity of pain and the effect of that pain on the individual. Nurses, by virtue of their role, spend proportionately more time with the patient than any other healthcare professional and they have a pivotal role to play in the accurate assessment of the patient's pain experience. It must be remembered, however, that pain assessment is a multidisciplinary activity and must go hand in hand with a thorough medical examination and investigation into the possible causes of pain.

The key to a good assessment is regularity. It is not a 'one off' intervention, but is part of a continuous process and failure to do this can result in the under treatment of the patient in pain. It is fair to say that research that has looked at the assessment of pain in many clinical environments and across many cultures has consistently shown that not only do patients underreport their pain for many different reasons, but even when it is reported nurses and medical staff often do not take the patient's pain seriously, and consequently that pain remains poorly managed (Farrer, 2007).

No profession holds a moral high ground here and it is a key objective of the World Health Organization to offer advice, support and information to any health professional involved in the assessment and management of pain in whatever environment (WHO, 2007).

What goes into pain assessment?

As pain is a subjective, personal experience the physical, psychological, social and environmental factors must all be considered as they influence the way in which people express and experience pain. The relationship between the different factors must also be explored in order to identify if the physical pain, for example, has induced psychological, and/or social problems or vice versa. The concept of total pain, which was explored in Chapter 8, will give you an idea of the kind of areas to explore.

The pain assessment interview

This is probably the most important area of all, and questions and observations done well at this point will help to give a very clear picture to the whole caring team. Conversations with people who are in pain are, by their very nature, emotive and potentially intense. It is vital therefore that a structure be adopted by the nurse or health professional so that when facilitating the patient's story of their pain a clear and comprehensive picture can be steadily built that reflects the patient's perceived priorities and allows for the prescription of a suitable regime to control the pain. This chapter will focus on the core elements that go into pain assessment.

Begin your assessment by looking at the patient. Look for non-verbal cues that suggest pain, for example body posture and facial expression. Although visual and verbal pain assessment tools are really very simple to use, they rely on the person being able to give a coherent response and take little account of those who may be cognitively impaired or whose consciousness level is fluctuating. This is why keen observation skills are so important.

Much of your pain assessment will revolve around a series of questions. Questioning should take place in a conversational style rather than an interrogation. It is not essential to ask all questions in one 'sitting'. The aim of pain assessment is to gather as much information about the patient's pain as possible. Don't forget to ask all the team members who have had contact with the patient about the patient's pain. Professionals such as physiotherapists and social workers may have something to add. So too may the home support workers and domestic staff.

Suggested questions:

- Would you like to tell me about your pain?
- What words do you use to describe your pain?
- Can you show me where it hurts?
- Is the pain there all the time?
- How long have you had this pain?
- Does the pain go anywhere else?
- What makes the pain better?
- What makes the pain worse?
- What medications are you taking for the pain?
- Do they help?
- Are you taking them as your doctor prescribed? (If not, why not?)
- Are you taking any medications your doctor did not prescribe? For example ibuprofen you bought from the supermarket?
- How do you feel about taking strong painkillers?
- Is there anything else you would like to tell me about your pain?

These questions are not definitive, nor are they designed to be asked in a particular order. Only you will know and understand the constraints and opportunities that make up the dynamics of the pain interview in your work environment. You will notice that some of the questions are closed and directive – to allow the patient to give you a short precise response. Other questions are more open and designed to elicit a conversational response to allow you to explore how the patient feels about *their* pain and to tell *their* story as *they* see it.

 Reflective activity

The next time you are on duty take with you a list of these questions and try some of them out on one of your patients who you know has pain that is now well controlled. Be careful to choose someone who you know well and ask their permission to talk to them about their pain. Choose a time of day that does not take you away from essential care activities and allow yourself around 15–30 minutes for this interview. Take down notes as you go along. Reread these notes a short while after the interview and ask yourself whether you have learned anything new that may inform the care of this patient. The chances are you will have.

Feedback: The benefit of doing an exercise such as this is that it can give you confidence to try out the pain interview in a situation that is more calm and settled first, so that there is no need to rush things and instigate emergency prescriptions to control bad pain. Among the things you may have picked up were issues around:

- How effective the medication currently is
- What times of the day are worse and which are better and why
- What strategies the person uses to alleviate their pain beyond the medication
- How they feel about the situation they are in
- Social, relationship, home and job issues that may be impinging on the pain

If it helps to have a structure to your assessment then consider a simple framework such as the one below:

- **Look and listen**: What are the main issues for this person? Some pains are more bearable than others and they may well point out a number of issues in their life that go along with the pain.
- **Consider the person's age, cultural background and ability to respond**: Children don't have the vocabulary to express their needs in the same way as adults and are usually very direct. Culture can play a large part in the perception of pain but beware of stereotypes. Those who are cognitively impaired may find it difficult to communicate verbally.
- **Listen actively to the problems in the patient's order of priority**: The patient's quality of life issues may be very different from how you perceive them regarding their pain.
- **Think of possible causes**: As your interview progresses you begin to get a better picture of what is happening.
- **Use assessment tools to help**: There are a selection of simple, pragmatic ones available which suit most situations. Decide on what works and is acceptable to your work area and make sure they are used by everyone involved.
- **Explore options**: Using the patient's agenda look at the different options available to you to help this person. Consider the elements of total pain as you look at these options. For example:

- – Feelings of helplessness can be alleviated by providing them with more opportunities to be involved in decision making about care.
- – Uncertainty can be helped by the offer of information when it is required in a way that can be understood.
- – Disturbed sleep can be helped by looking at the patient's routine and offering strategies to promote a regular sleep pattern.
- **Plan**: Agree with the person the way forward, document this and inform those members of the team who need to know.
- **Explain**: To family members what is happening if appropriate and the patient wishes it so.
- **Review**: Pain changes continually so nursing and medical care must be reviewed regularly for its effectiveness in controlling pain. How often you do this will depend on the resources available to you, but ideally every 24 hours until the pain is well controlled.

The barriers to pain assessment

For pain to be accurately assessed and thereby appropriately managed all health professionals must be aware of the potential barriers to pain assessment.

Those associated with the patient and family include:

- A belief that pain is inevitable and untreatable
- Failure to contact the appropriate medical services
- 'Putting on a brave face' to the health professionals
- Not taking the prescribed medication due to a suspicion of or non-belief in the efficacy of modern drugs
- A belief that you should only take the medication if it's absolutely necessary
- Non-compliance due to the fear of addiction
- Non-compliance due to the fear that tolerance will rapidly develop leaving nothing left for when the pain gets really bad
- Stopping medication because of adverse side effects and not telling the professionals
- Religious beliefs regarding suffering and pain
- Fixed and narrow beliefs about pain medication based on gossip, media portrayals and cultural myths

Those associated with health professionals include:

- Ignoring the patient's pain believing it to be inevitable and untreatable

- Unawareness of the intensity of the patient's pain
- A failure to get behind the 'brave face'
- The medication prescribed is too weak to relieve the pain
- Failure to give the patient adequate instructions about the use of analgesics
- Not establishing a joint strategy of care with the patient, the family and other professionals
- Not monitoring progress often enough
- Poor knowledge base and attitude of the professionals and a reluctance to ask for help
- Fixed and narrow beliefs about pain medication based on gossip, media portrayals and cultural myths

On a wider note there are a number of other significant factors which also impede a successful pain assessment:

- The lack of a clearly defined language of pain that is understood worldwide
- Anxiety, depression, young children, cognitive impairment or any disability that reduces the person's ability to clearly communicate their pain
- Environmental constraints such as noise, light, heat or cold

The reality of pain assessment

There are many useful pain assessment tools in existence and the golden rules are that the tools must be simple to use for the patient and professional. (Remember these tools are only as good as how the professional uses them, so don't go straight to the tools before you allow the patient to tell their story.)

Rating scales

These ask the patient to give their pain a numerical or verbal rating – for example a score out of ten with 0 = no pain and 10 = the worst pain imaginable. While these scales are helpful please remember that pain is a highly subjective experience that is difficult to reduce to a number. Many patients find pain scales difficult to use.

A numerical pain scale

A numerical pain scale (Figure 9.1) allows you to describe the intensity of your discomfort in numbers ranging from 0 to 10 (or greater depending on the scale).

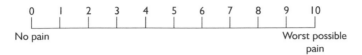

Figure 9.1 A numerical pain scale (taken from McCaffery and Pasero, 1999).

A verbal pain scale

With a verbal pain scale (Figure 9.2) the degree of discomfort is described by choosing one of the vertical lines that most corresponds to the intensity of pain the person is feeling. This scale can determine if recovery is progressing in a positive direction.

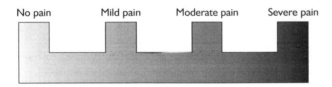

Figure 9.2 A verbal pain scale.

The Wong–Baker Faces Pain Rating Scale (Figure 9.3; Wong *et al.*, 2001) is designed for children aged 3 years and older and is also helpful for elderly patients and those who may be cognitively impaired.

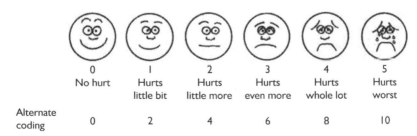

Figure 9.3 The Wong–Baker Faces Pain Rating Scale.

Each face shows how a person in pain is feeling.

Body outlines

These (Figure 9.4) allow the user to indicate where the pains are experienced. Ask the patient to show you where the pains are and either mark this on the chart yourself or better still get the patient to do so if that is appropriate. It takes very little time to do and can help greatly when the cause of the pain is being diagnosed.

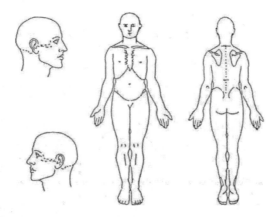

Figure 9.4 Body outlines pain assessment.

Pain diaries

These can be very useful with difficult pain, where it is hard to get a complete picture of what is happening. Some patients may find it useful to keep a diary about their pain. A simple format will suffice like the one suggested below.

Date	Time	Pain score (0–5)	Activity	Comments
Monday	09:00	4	Getting dressed	Hurts when I bend
Monday	09:45	2	Resting	Took morphine
Monday	11:40	1	Talked to GP	Really helped
Monday	13:00	5	Walking, windy day	Pain in face V bad. Took pink medicine
Monday	15:00	0	Sleeping	
Monday	17:30	2	Eating tea	Pain behind breast bone

The action of keeping a diary can be empowering for some but tedious for others. The main benefit of this record is that it provides an opportunity to promote discussion about when the pain is worse and, more positively, what helps to alleviate the pain. Adjustments to the medications and other management strategies can then be used to help the patient at these difficult times.

Whatever tool and assessment approach is used it is essential that you record your findings for others to use. A seemingly insignificant comment may provide useful clues in the management of a complex pain.

For those of you who wish to utilise a more systematic and detailed approach to pain assessment there are a small selection of validated and reliable pain assessment tools that are available, for example:

- Memorial Pain Assessment Card (Fishman *et al.*, 1987). A simple, rapidly completed questionnaire which measures intensity, relief of pain and psychological distress. Developed for use in hospitals.
- Wisconsin Brief Pain Inventory (Daut *et al.*, 1983). Widely used across many cultures to assess pain. It measures the intensity and relief of pain, psychological distress and functional impairment and is a valid and reliably tested tool used in research studies. A shortened version has been used in research and in the hospice setting.
- McGill Pain Questionnaire (Melzack, 1993). One of the first pain assessment tools, which revolutionised assessment in this area. The full chart is very detailed and time consuming to complete, but a shortened version is available. Still used actively in research.

Reflective activity

This activity is similar to the one earlier in this chapter.

The next time you are on duty take with you a copy of one or more of the assessment tools on offer and try them out on two of your patients who you know have pain that is now well controlled. Be careful to choose someone who you know well and ask their permission to talk to them about their pain experience over the previous few days. Choose a time of day that does not take you away from essential care activities and allow yourself around 15–30 minutes for this interview. Take down notes as you go along. Re-read these notes a short while after the interview and ask yourself whether you have learnt anything new that may inform the care of these patients. The chances are you will have.

Feedback: The benefit of doing an exercise such as this is that it will help give you confidence in the use of pain assessment tools in a situation that is more calm and settled first, so that there is no need to rush things and instigate emergency prescriptions to control bad pain. Among the things you may have picked up were issues around:

- What times of the day are worse and which times are better and why
- Which tool is best suited to which person
- How the scoring is different for each person even though they may describe their pain in a similar way

Case study application

Judith and family: background information

This married couple are both 46 years old and live in a small housing estate on the edge of town. John is a labourer and is often out of work, whilst Judith has a part time job at a local clothing factory. Their son Christopher (9) is a bright but quiet lad who is very close to his father. John and his son share a love of fishing and spend most weekends at the local lake. The family are practising Christians. Judith was married before to Tom, who lives nearby with their two teenage children from this marriage (Henry 12, and Nikki 14) and his new wife. They all get on reasonably well, but the two elder children sometimes behave badly towards Christopher.

They are a close, trusting and caring family who have few friends and lead a very private life. Judith has an old school friend (Cheryl) who is a trusted confidante, living a few doors away, but John is very much a loner. He is the main decision maker, who sees himself as the traditional head of the family, and Judith has a rather nervous disposition and is inclined to panic at times over relatively minor things. Judith's elderly mother died six months ago after a long illness. She lived a long way from their home and Judith could not provide the support she wanted for her because of the distance. John's family emigrated many years prior and he has no contact with them.

Recently Judith has been feeling unwell and has not been eating properly. She has had a lot of indigestion and heartburn and eventually went to her family doctor. He sent her for investigations and an epigastric mass was found. The consultant decided to get her into hospital as soon as possible for an exploratory laparotomy. A huge gastric tumour was found with extensive liver and pelvic deposits with bone involvement. The surgeons closed her up with no procedure done.

Judith's pain

She was given some pethidine post-operatively which was successful in controlling her pain over the first 12–24 hours. It is now five days since the surgery and she continues to be nauseous throughout the day.

Her abdominal pain, however, is steadily getting worse and is radiating down her back. It is constant and she can only get some comfort by curling into the foetal position, which she maintains for hours at a time. Her mood is now low and she communicates little to the staff. She is uncomplaining of pain, but her facial expressions, mannerisms and behaviour suggest otherwise. The night staff say that she is crying a lot in the early hours. The hospital chaplain has been to see her, and her parish vicar. She seems to get some comfort from their visits, but voices are sometimes raised in anger and they leave soon after. She has also started complaining of headaches and gastritis, which seem to get worse before she has a visit from her family or the doctor. She wants to go home as soon as possible, but is concerned about whether her family will be able to cope and tries hard to convince the team that her pain is much better and she will be okay.

 Reflective activity

In terms of her holistic pain what would be your assessment of this situation?

Feedback: In your interview with Judith it is important to be guided by her agenda, which will inevitably involve trying to convince you that she is not suffering much pain and is able to go home. However, here we have a situation where the Mc-Caffery (1983) definition of pain ('pain is what the experiencing person says it is, existing whenever he says it does') could be challenged. Judith's priority to go home has to be balanced against her answers to your questions and your and the team's observations of Judith's body language and behaviour throughout the day, coupled with any information her family may be able to supply you. Only then will you be able to get a full picture of her pain. Note that two of her pains are *not* caused by her cancer.

If we use the framework for the pain assessment interview suggested earlier on in this chapter, this is the kind of result we may come up with.

- **Look and listen**: The main issues for Judith centre around getting herself well enough to go home to her family for the last period of her life. Her conversation will be dominated by this, so it's important we listen carefully and acknowledge the reality of her pain experience.
- **Consider the person's age, cultural background and ability to respond**: Judith is still a young woman at 46 and is having to face the prospect of not seeing any of her children grow up, or of fulfilling a long relationship with her husband. Although she is a private lady she is also known to be an anxious person and this should be borne in mind when talking to her. Trust is important for someone like her, and your skills at developing a rapport with her will help you to get some honest replies regarding her pain. Let's not forget that she has a strong personal faith which may give her immense spiritual support, or

be severely challenged by this illness. This aspect of your holistic assessment should be done with care and sensitivity.

- **Listen actively to the problems in the patient's order of priority**: Judith will in part be guided by yourself and the questions you ask, but she will also have certain key priorities which need to be noted. Her quality of life issues may be very different from how you perceive them regarding her pain.
- **Think of possible causes**: As your interview progresses with Judith you begin to get a better picture of what the holistic nature of her pain is, and causes may well spring to mind quite quickly. Resist the temptation to hijack the interview at this point, but make sure you note down those causes to come back to later. As well as the more obvious physical pains, don't forget the psycho-social element, for example:
  - Fear of losing control over her life and independence. Worries over her son Christopher and his future and the difficult relationship with Henry and Nikki who may feel shut out. Anxiety regarding the home and financial security.
- **Use assessment tools to help**: The numerical, verbal and pictorial pain scales are all appropriate to use with Judith in your assessment. It may also be useful for the staff to keep a diary of her pain over 24 hours. (Normally it would be Judith who would keep a diary, but bearing in mind her behaviour and her goal to go home as soon as possible, she is likely to not be honest in her reporting.) An accurate assessment of the nature of these pains will enable you to work out a number of strategies to help her both in the immediate short term and longer term.
- **Explore options**: This is the key part of the management of her pain and will be covered in detail in Chapter 10.
- **Plan**: Once Judith, her family and the team have agreed the way forward then the management can begin. Clear and up-to-date documentation of your assessment of her pain and the subsequent management strategy is vital. Make sure that all the relevant team members are aware.
- **Explain**: Judith's husband will almost certainly want to know the outcome of your assessment. It is normally good practice to ask Judith's permission first before telling him, but this depends on the cultural norms within your health-care system.
- **Review**: If the management strategy is effective then Judith's pain will alter radically over the next 24 hours. In the first instance it would be appropriate to review her pain after 1–2 hours and 6 hourly thereafter. After 24 hours it will depend on the resources you have available (i.e. drug availability and support systems) but ideally once a day until her pain is well controlled.

The skills required to assess pain

Just how competent are you to assess pain and how do you know that the skills you have developed are based around a sound evidence base? Work from people like Benner (1984) who writes about nurses moving from 'novice to expert' on a continuum provides us with a clear idea of the ways in which adults learn in the 'real world' of practice.

If you have attempted the activities in this chapter and in Chapter 8 you will already have a good level of knowledge. Such activities are useful to consolidate learning and this kind of reflective process is very useful, but the ability to think and write effectively does not necessarily translate into competence in clinical skills. This is why it is important that we take an honest and critical look at our perceived level of skills in pain assessment so that we can work towards improving our practice.

One way of doing this is to undertake a self-assessment using competency statements. They are designed to be a means by which you can obtain a baseline assessment of your clinical skills in pain assessment in your work environment and will help you identify deficits in areas that need to be addressed and also help you to acknowledge skills that are already well developed. There is a simple three-category graduated scale used to enable you to make your decision as you work your way through the document.

What is a competency?

There are numerous definitions available for the term competency, but for our purposes we will concentrate on the definition cited by the RCN in relation to specialist palliative nursing (RCN, 2002, p. 2). Competence in a given set of skills can be defined as

> The skills, knowledge, experience, attributes and behaviours required by an individual in order to perform the job effectively.

In order to work, therefore, it relies on the formulation of agreed competency statements that are then identified at differing levels of practice.

What are the levels of practice?

- **Explored**: To examine and investigate systematically an area or skill related to practice.

- **Practised**: To take a skill and use it appropriately in the clinical area on a repeated basis.
- **Developed**: To progress in the knowledge, application and evaluation of a skill and demonstrate this in practice.

This scale has been taken and adapted from the generic assessment tool in palliative nursing devised by Becker (2000).

What do I do?

1. Read the competency statements thoroughly and familiarise yourself with the grading structure.
2. Set some time aside to conduct your own self-assessment of your current skills level (p. 167). This will help you to identify areas for development, which can be addressed in your clinical practice.
3. It is helpful if you can select perhaps 2–3 competencies that are priorities; these can then be written into a learning contract (p. 168) to help you focus on what needs to be done to move your skills forward (a suggested format for a learning contract is offered to you). The real learning and development rests upon your ability to examine the deficits and plan a strategy to deal with these issues in your everyday practice.

This process has the added advantage of clarifying and validating to you what you perceive you are already competent at, where this is evident. This is important to our professional development, as sometimes it can be difficult to acknowledge and articulate what we know we are good at in our job when the culture of nursing is so often centred on identifying the problems rather than the achievements.

The success of this approach lies very much in your ability to be both honest and reflective in your assessment. It is undoubtedly challenging both intellectually and personally to put one's perceived skills so closely under scrutiny, but if we are to improve the care of those in pain in whatever setting it takes place, then it is important to define clearly what it is we expect a nurse to do and at what standard. The evidence base presented by this competency process is but one small step in this direction and is offered to you as an opportunity to engage in such work.

Pain assessment competencies

	Explored	Practised	Developed
1. Demonstrate and articulate an active commitment to the holistic assessment of pain			
2. Apply knowledge of the nature of pain to the assessment of that pain			
3. Discuss the concept of total pain and its relevance to patient-centred care in a palliative context			
4. Explore the implications for practice of individual perception and expression of pain			
5. Acknowledge the all pervading experience of total pain on the patient, family and carer			
6. Conduct a pain assessment interview using a range of available frameworks and tools			
7. Regularly review the pain assessment to enable an effective pain management strategy			
8. Recognise situations where a range of alternative strategies and psychological and spiritual support can be of benefit to the patient in the assessment and control of total pain			
9. Explore the concepts of patient autonomy relating to pain assessment			
10. Demonstrate competency in the assessment of total pain			

Consolidating your learning

Now that you have actively taken the time to examine your skills level, and hopefully worked on a strategy to improve your pain assessment skills, you will need to consolidate your learning.

It can be helpful to revisit your original assessment and to rescore yourself after a period of time (p. 169). (It is suggested that you may need a week or two to do this, but it is entirely dependent on your individual circumstances.)

Suggested learning contract

Identified pain assessment competency:

Self-assessment rating:
Explored ☐   **Practised** ☐   **Developed** ☐

Resources and Strategies (What do I need to do to improve my competency level?)

Evidence of Accomplishment (How can I demonstrate what I have learnt?)

Target Date: ....

Criteria for validating skills accomplishment:

How do you now judge your skill in this competency?

Explored ☐   **Practised** ☐   **Developed** ☐

	Your original score			Your score now		
	Explored	Practised	Developed	Explored	Practised	Developed
1. Demonstrate and articulate an active commitment to the holistic assessment of pain						
2. Apply knowledge of the nature of pain to the assessment of that pain						
3. Discuss the concept of total pain and its relevance to patient-centred care in a palliative context						
4. Explore the implications for practice of individual perception and expression of pain						
5. Acknowledge the all pervading experience of total pain on the patient, family and carer						
6. Conduct a pain assessment interview using a range of available frameworks and tools						
7. Regularly review the pain assessment to enable an effective pain management strategy						
8. Recognise situations where a range of alternative strategies and psychological and spiritual support can be of benefit to the patient in the assessment and control of total pain						
9. Explore the concepts of patient autonomy relating to pain assessment						
10. Demonstrate competency in the assessment of total pain						

Reflective activity

Try to answer the next few questions and keep a note of your responses:

- Some of your scores may have moved right across the scale and others not moved at all. Write down a few notes as to why this is so and what helped or hindered you in your attempts to improve your pain assessment skills?
- In an exercise like this there are nearly always things that you have done that on reflection you would have done differently. Write down what these are and what it is you will do differently next time.
- What insights have you gained about your own skills in pain assessment? For example:
  - Were you surprised at how good you were?
  - Were you surprised at how bad you were?
  - Did you expose your knowledge limitations and feel awkward at times?
  - Did you find out things about your patients that surprised you?
  - Did it confirm what you already knew?
- This is the difficult part. Now write down three things that you have learnt that you are able to take back to your practice.

Conclusion

In this chapter we have taken a comprehensive look at the assessment of pain and suffering as understood from the patient's lived experience. The good news is pain assessment does not require complex and expensive equipment and resources and can be utilised in almost any caring environment. It does, however, require a regular commitment and a holistic approach that moves beyond the medical model that dominates care today. This is the real challenge for all staff, but the potential benefits for our patients are enormous.

Your study so far will give you a clearer comprehension of the complex nature of pain assessment and will hopefully stimulate your thinking and cause you to reflect on your own practice, wherever that may be. The next step is to look at how we can take this knowledge and apply it to the management of pain in Chapter 10.

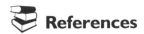 **References**

Benner, P. (1984) *From Novice to Expert: Excellence and Power in Clinical Practice.* Addison-Wesley, California.

Becker, R. (2000) Competency assessment in palliative nursing. *European Journal of Palliative Care*, **7**(3), 88–91.

Becker, R. and Gamlin, R. (2004) *Fundamental Aspects of Palliative Care Nursing.* Quay Books, Salisbury.

Carper, B. (1978) Fundamental patterns of knowing in nursing. *Advances in Nursing Science*, **1**(v), 13–23.

Daut, R. L., Cleeland, C. S. and Flanery, R. C. (1983) Development of the Wisconsin Brief Pain Questionnaire to assess pain in cancer and other diseases. *Pain*, **17**, 197–210.

Elliott, B. A., Elliott, T. E., Murray, D. M., Braun, B. L. and Johnson, K. M. (1996) Patients and family members: the role of knowledge and attitudes in cancer pain. *Journal of Pain Symptom Management*, **12**, 209–20.

Farrer, K. (2007) Pain control. In *Palliative Nursing: Improving End of Life Care*, 2nd edn (eds. S. Kinghorn and S. Gaines). Baillière-Tindall, Ediinburgh.

Field, L. (1996) Are nurses still underestimating patients' pain postoperatively? *British Journal of Nursing*, **13**, 778–84.

Fishman, B., Pasternak, S., Wallenstein, S. L., Houde, R. W., Holland, J. C. and Foley, K. M. (1987) The Memorial Pain Assessment Card. A valid instrument for the evaluation of cancer pain. *Cancer*, **60**, 1151–8.

McCaffery, M. (1983). *Nursing the Patient in Pain.* Harper & Row, London.

McCaffery, M. and Pasero, C. (1999). *Pain Clinical Manual*, 2nd edn, p. 63. Mosby, St Louis.

Melzack, R. (1993) The McGill Pain Questionnaire. In *Pain Measurement and Assessment* (ed. R. Melzack), pp. 41–8. Raven Press, New York.

Royal College of Nursing (2002) *A Framework for Nurses Working in Specialist Palliative Care: Competencies Project.* RCN Publications, London.

Wong, D. L. (2001). *Wong's Essentials of Paediatric Nursing*, 6th edn, p. 1301. Mosby, St Louis.

World Health Organization (2007) *Cancer Pain Release.* http://www.whocancerpain. wisc.edu/contents.html. Accessed 6 July 2007.

Original material for this chapter was taken and adapted from the Assessment of Pain online study course authored by R. Becker and available at the following reference:

http://www.cancernursing.org/

 Useful websites

Scottish Intercollegiate Guidelines Network – pain control
http://www.sign.ac.uk/guidelines/fulltext/44/

Pain.com
http://www.pain.com/sections/categories_of_pain/cancer/

Cancer pain.org
http://www.cancer-pain.org/

Cancer pain management in children
http://www.childcancerpain.org/

Hospice Net
http://www.hospicenet.org/html/what_is_pain.html

The Oxford Pain internet Site
http://www.jr2.ox.ac.uk/bandolier/booth/painpag/

📋 Chapter links to the Nursing and Midwifery Council Standards of Conduct, Performance and Ethics for Nurses and Midwives (2008)

Section 1: Make the care of people your first concern, treating them as individuals and respecting their dignity

Treat people as individuals
- You must treat people as individuals and respect their dignity
- You must treat people kindly and considerately
- You must act as an advocate for those in your care, helping them to access relevant health and social care, information and support

Collaborate with those in your care
- You must listen to the people in your care and respond to their concerns and preferences
- You must support people in caring for themselves to improve and maintain their health
- You must recognise and respect the contribution that people make to their own care and wellbeing
- You must make arrangements to meet people's language and communication needs
- You must share with people, in a way they can understand, the information they want or need to know about their health

Section 2: Work with others to protect and promote the health and wellbeing of those in your care, their families and carers, and the wider community

Share information with your colleagues
■ You must keep your colleagues informed when you are sharing the care of others

Work effectively as part of a team
■ You must work cooperatively within teams and respect the skills, expertise and contributions of your colleagues
■ You must consult and take advice from colleagues when appropriate
■ You must make a referral to another practitioner when it is in the best interests of someone in your care

Section 3: Provide a high standard of practice and care at all times

Use the best available evidence
■ You must deliver care based on the best available evidence or best practice.

Keep your skills and knowledge up to date
■ You must have the knowledge and skills for safe and effective practice when working without direct supervision
■ You must recognise and work within the limits of your competence
■ You must take part in appropriate learning and practice activities that maintain and develop your competence and performance

Keep clear and accurate records
■ You must keep clear and accurate records of the discussions you have, the assessments you make, the treatment and medicines you give and how effective these have been
■ You must complete records as soon as possible after an event has occurred
■ You must not tamper with original records in any way
■ You must ensure any entries you make in someone's paper records are clearly and legibly signed, dated and timed
■ You must ensure any entries you make in someone's electronic records are clearly attributable to you
■ You must ensure all records are kept confidentially and securely

☑ Self-assessment test

1. A pain assessment scale is used to:
   A   Measure pain intensity
   B   Evaluate character of pain
   C   Monitor compliance with medication regimen
   D   Measure cultural differences in perceiving pain

2. After each assessment, pain should be reviewed every:
   A   12–24 hours
   B   24–48 hours
   C   48–72 hours

3. Body outlines allow the user to:
   A   Describe the discomfort by choosing a vertical line
   B   Describe the discomfort numerically
   C   Indicate where the discomfort is experienced

4 Using a structure to your questioning in the assessment interview can help you to:
   A   Build up a clear picture of the pain
   B   Look at options for better management
   C   Consider other factors such as age or culture
   D   All of the above

5. Which of these statements regarding barriers to pain assessment is true?
   A   Pain is inevitable and untreatable
   B   You should only take your medication if absolutely necessary
   C   There's no point putting on a 'brave face'; it's better to tell the nurse how bad it really is
   D   If I take too much then I will become addicted

CHAPTER 10

The management of pain

 Jim asked for oxygen – his worsening condition was making him restless. Suddenly a central crushing pain: a 10 on the scale and getting worse he said. Staff calmly gave the right medication, checked his vital signs, brought a fan to his bedside, and sat quietly with him, reassuring him from time to time. Soon all was calm again and with his wife by his side Jim drifted in and out of consciousness. There were no loud buzzers, no calls for 'crash' and racing around, just expert care and compassion delivered with dignity. Why can't pain always be managed with such skill?

Learning outcomes

After reading this chapter and completing the reflective activities the learner will be able to:

■ Understand the goals and principles that underpin the management of total pain in a palliative care context
■ Clarify the reality of pain management from the myths that exist in many environments
■ Appreciate the need for a multi-professional and holistic approach in the management of chronic pain
■ Describe the core skills of the nurse in the management of chronic pain
■ Assess and reflect on your competency in pain management by using the tools offered

In this chapter we will take a comprehensive look at the management of pain and suffering as understood from the patient's lived experience and applied to nursing practice. Whilst it is recognised that in most countries in the world the prescription of major opiate drugs to control chronic nociceptive pain is the direct responsibility of the doctor, it is the nurse who often has to deliver these drugs and many others besides and monitor the patient's progress. It is the nurse who supports and reassures the patient and family and often helps to dispel the myths surrounding the use of opiates, which in turn helps to ensure compliance and therefore good pain control.

175

It is also nurses who, by the very nature of their caring philosophy, are naturally oriented towards holistic thinking and embrace the tenets of 'total pain' much more readily than many medical staff. This helps to ensure that the psychosocial, spiritual and emotional elements are seen as equal partners in the management of chronic pain.

It is not just pharmacology that can help to relieve pain. If you have studied the previous two chapters (8 and 9) you will know already that there are a number of highly effective strategies that can be adopted to complement a medically prescribed drug regime. Indeed, as you will discover, there are many pains which will respond well to the creative, compassionate responses of an interested and caring nurse.

The concept of 'total pain' which was explored in the previous chapter will give us a clear idea of what needs to be looked at when devising a pain management strategy. This is where the art and science of good palliative care come together in perhaps the most practical and useful way to ease suffering.

The barriers to pain management

No matter how knowledgeable and proficient a practitioner may be, there are nearly always a range of factors that can get in the way of utilising a successful pain management strategy. Some of these are intrinsic to the work environment and beyond our control to change, but there are many others which are rooted in ignorance, prejudice, tradition and attitude that are within our power to influence. Make no mistake, the challenging of behaviours and attitudes that are ingrained custom and practice is not easy and requires determination, resilience and courage. If successful, however, your patients will thank you for it.

It is appropriate therefore, that before we take a look at the frameworks which can help us manage pain we take a step back and acknowledge these barriers, so that we can reflect on how much they affect our work and whether our own attitudes and behaviours need to be challenged.

Healthcare professionals

The availability of education for those who need expertise in pain management varies hugely around the world. In most western countries with a well-developed healthcare infrastructure there are many opportunities available for healthcare staff to access such education. It should be expected therefore, that the standard of pain control is high in the West, but the statistics for cancer in particular, are not good. We may have the science to control 90% of cancer pain, but this is not reflected in clinical practice (Pargeon and Hailey, 1999).

The reasons for this are many. Doctors fear litigation if they over-prescribe controlled drugs such as opiates and there is a fear of addiction and analgesic tolerance. Furthermore, there is a general lack of awareness in some countries that pain can be adequately controlled. Negative media representations of the misuse of morphine have also contributed to restrictive and misguided legislation reducing the availability of major opiates in places where they are desperately needed (WHO, 1990).

Patients and family members

All cultures differ in their knowledge, attitudes and behaviours towards pain as a lived experience, and by far the most common reasons for poor pain relief include fear of addiction, fear of side effects, fear of drug tolerance and lack of knowledge. Sometimes the recognition of severe pain and the advanced disease that is causing it is psychologically unacceptable, because that means recognising that death may be imminent and therefore consciously foregoing hope for recovery. This deeply ingrained attitude is prevalent in a number of cultures who see active medical curative measures as entirely appropriate up to the moment of death. The concept of futility, as those in the West would understand, it is therefore not acknowledged.

Adverse side effects may also cause people to stop taking effective medication and there may also be a non-belief in the efficacy of modern drugs. In some cultures there is the very real belief that pain is inevitable and the person must 'suffer in silence'. As a result there are an unknown number of people with advanced disease and chronic pain who never get to see a doctor.

Cost issues should also be acknowledged as a significant factor in enabling patients and families to access what drugs are available. Restrictive government legislation creates shortages and prices rise accordingly. In developing countries many families cannot afford to purchase the required drugs even if they are available.

The analgesic ladder

In 1982 the World Health Organization approached a panel of experts and asked them to devise a simple and understandable approach for the management of pain. What they came up with has been called the 'analgesic ladder' (Figure 10.1). This ladder is a simple, reliable and effective way to under-

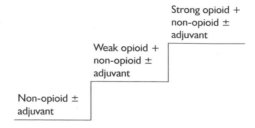

Figure 10.1 Pharmacological management of pain: the World Health Organization analgesic ladder (WHO, 1986, 1996).

stand the pharmacological management of chronic pain. In those countries experienced in its use there has been a review of its structure and a number of physicians now question the need for the second level; however, for those resource-poor countries whose access to drugs is severely limited by financial, attitudinal and socio-political factors the three-stage ladder remains the mainstay approach to use. For a fascinating review of the WHO analgesic ladder see Porta-Sales *et al.* (2003).

The ladder explained

The methodology is simple and involves a stepwise approach to the use of analgesic drugs, moving from the first to the third step in stages according to the strength of the analgesic drugs needed.

Step One
Patients are treated with non-opioid analgesics such as paracetamol, aspirin or non-steroidal anti-inflammatory drugs such as ibuprofen or diclofenac (NSAIDs). Adverse effects such as gastric irritation and peptic ulceration are common with NSAIDs. Many patients will respond well to regular doses of step one drugs.

Step Two
Patients with moderate pain who are not pain-free on Step One should be treated with a weak opioid drug together with other drugs as necessary. Weak opioids include codeine, dihydrocodeine, dextropopoxyphene and tramadol. You will be familiar with co-codamol, a mixture of paracetamol and codeine, and co-dydramol, which combines paracetamol and dihydrocodeine. These drugs are effective and very commonly prescribed.

Step Three

Patients experiencing severe pain or those who are not pain-free on Step Two should receive a strong analgesic. If necessary this can be combined with non-opioid drugs which are often called adjuvants. Strong opioids include morphine, diamorphine and fentanyl. Alternative opioids exist for example, hydromorphone, methadone and oxycodone. It is essential to consult a pain specialist or palliative care specialist before prescribing alternative opioids.

Divided opinion

There is a growing body of opinion today that the division of analgesic drugs into the 'weak' and 'strong' is arbitrary and at times the wrong way to think. For example, the use of full doses of weak opioids at Step Two represents the same as a small dose of strong opioids in terms of its efficacy (Porta-Sales *et al.*, 2003). For many resource-poor countries in the world, where strong opioids are either not available or restricted, this is a more realistic perspective.

Remember that controlling pain via the ladder can happen in both directions. For example, if a person needs a strong analgesic to gain control of their pain in the first instance, it is possible that once things have stabilised the type or strength of the analgesic can be reduced. When using analgesic drugs remember that the severity of pain on its own does not give enough information to choose analgesics. Not every patient will require strong opioids. They should never be used as euphoriants or sedatives for instance, to elevate the mood or to sedate.

Not all pains are very sensitive to opioids. If the pain is partially sensitive or not sensitive to opioids, then consider adjuvant drugs or additional analgesics; other methods, such as transcutaneous electrical nerve stimulation (TENS), nerve blocks or spinal procedures, can be helpful. All of the above suggestions depend entirely on the availability of such resources in your work environment, and where these resources do not exist perhaps the best advice is to always contact the nearest palliative care specialist so that a suitable strategy can be agreed. There is always something that can be done.

It is important for the team to think about treatable causes of pain. For example, radiotherapy can be used to treat bone metastasis, and surgery may fix a long bone that is about to fracture.

🖉 Reflective activity

Take a look at the range of analgesics available to you in your work area and make yourself a list. Next, try to categorise these into the steps of the ladder and you will begin to get an idea of where the gaps are and where you can maximise pain control through the creative use of the ladder to give combinations of drugs that can control pain.

The golden rules for pain control

There are a few simply understood and widely accepted principles that under-pin the prescription of pain-relieving medication. The good news is that they are easy to remember and can be cited in clinical practice to support care.

The first principles were devised by the WHO (WHO, 1986,1996) as part of the work that went into the development of the analgesic ladder. They are:

- **By the mouth**: Oral administration is the first route of choice for the admin-istration of opioids including morphine. It is recognised, however, that in many countries morphine may only be available in injection form, due to restrictive legislation limiting the availability of oral morphine. Where any analgesic is available orally and the patient is capable of swallowing it, this is always the preferred route.
- **By the clock**: This emphasises the importance of preventative prescribing for chronic pain. Analgesics should always be given in sufficient doses and regularly enough firstly to control the pain and secondly to keep that pain at bay.
- **By the ladder**: Use the three-step analgesic ladder as your guide and move up appropriately according to the patient's response.

The following principles have no particular author and there are numer-ous variations in the content, but the messages are important and often cited as:

The 10 Commandments of Good Pain Control
1. Do not assume that the patient's pain is caused by the malignant process
2. Take the patient's feelings into consideration at all times
3. Do not use the abbreviation PRN (*pro re nata* – meaning 'as necessary')
4. Do not prescribe or endorse inadequate amounts of analgesia
5. Always try non-opiate analgesics in the first instance
6. Do not be afraid to use opiate analgesics
7. Do not limit your approach to simply analgesics
8. Do not be afraid to ask a colleague's advice
9. Always provide support for the whole family
10. Develop an air of quiet confidence and cautious optimism

The final principles that are often cited refer primarily to cancer pain management and embody some of what has been said already, but with some important extra components:

- Be aware that the pain may be due to the cancer and its treatment, but it may also be due to another pathology.
- Communicate all pain-related findings to the team.
- Observe patients carefully and anticipate. Don't wait for them to tell you they have pain.
- Assess pain meticulously and repeatedly.
- If pain is not controlled by proper doses of the drug at regular intervals, move up to the next level on the analgesic ladder.
- Review the efficacy of the dosage at regular intervals.
- If necessary increase the prescription by 25–50%.
- Use prescribed, individually adjusted, regular analgesia so that the pain does not return.
- Set realistic goals with the patient.
- There is no maximum dose for morphine or diamorphine
- Constipation is inevitable, so always prescribe a suitable laxative/stool softener.
- Nausea and vomiting occurs in half of patients, though usually only for 3–5 days. Anti-emetics can be useful in this phase.
- For patients in pain, addiction is never a problem.
- Respiratory depression is rarely seen in patients using opioids for chronic pain.
- Analgesic drugs alone will not relieve all pain. Compassion, empathy, understanding, diversion and elevation of mood are essential complementary measures.
- If you are not successful in managing pain go back to the concept of total pain and ask, 'What have I missed'?

Adapted and expanded from Regnard and Tempest (1998).

The pharmacological management of pain

The science of pain control has come a long way in the last fifty years and our understanding of the efficacy of a wide range of approaches has increased dramatically. Advances in the pharmacology associated with pain control have run in parallel to this and a clear understanding of the use of the major drugs in this area is vital to success. There is more to good pain control than simple prescribing, however, and there is need to look at the combinations of drugs that can constitute a suitable regime.

Routes of administration

There are many ways by which drugs can be administered to the body and the choice of route will depend on a number of factors. For those who live and work in resource-poor countries there may be no other choice than by injection ,as oral morphine is unavailable due to restrictive legislation. For those who work in countries where there are more resources there are a variety of options available.

The physical condition of the person may well be a factor in choice of route; e.g. the cachexic person may not be able to tolerate intramuscular, sub-cutaneous or intravenous routes due to muscle wastage, poor skin condition and collapsed veins. The cognitively impaired may benefit from drug adminis-tration via a skin patch. The person with pain caused by a tumour compressing the spinal cord will almost certainly benefit from drug administration given via the epidural route. It is useful therefore to take some time to look at exactly what the choices are, why they are used and their relative efficacy.

- **Oral**   Oral administration is always the first route of choice for the admin-istration of any pain-relieving medication where the person is capable of taking the drugs and resources exist to provide this option. It is also the easiest route for the patient and the cheapest in terms of the purchase of analgesics. This is an important issue and contentious for many practition-ers who work in developing countries, where the media portrayal of opiate misuse as a recreational drug has led to legislation that only allows the import of expensive opiate injections instead of the cheaper oral options, which actively disadvantages pain management for those who desperately need it.

  There are also no major complications with the oral choice. Mostly there are two types of formulation available: 'normal release' and 'slow release'. The slow release drugs have been formulated to give longer lasting pain relief and are usually given twice a day. The normal release formulations can be used to titrate opioid requirements against the pain and are useful for any breakthrough pain. Morphine, oxycodone and hydromorphone are all examples of major analgesics that are available in both formulations.

- **Transmucosal and sublingual**   This is where drugs are absorbed either through the lining of the mouth or under the tongue. These routes are useful for those patients who cannot tolerate oral medication due to nausea, vomiting or dysphagia. They can also be used for those who are emaciated and where their veins have collapsed. These routes are simple to use and because of the rapid absorption due to rich venous supply, there is quicker pain relief. Drugs such as methadone, fentanyl and buprenorphine are better absorbed sublingually, and a fentanyl lozenge exists for just this reason. The lozenge needs to be rubbed against the mucosa of the cheek rather than sucked and is used mostly for breakthrough pain. The main side effects of drugs used via these routes relate to the bitter taste in the mouth and sometimes a burning sensation.

- **Transdermal** This route is associated with absorption through the skin and has become very popular in recent years due to its non-invasive nature, and for those people who are unable or unwilling to take drugs orally this is a useful option to have.

  Fentanyl (an opioid analgesic) has been available for several years as a patch. It is useful in patients who have achieved good pain control with other opioids, and after application to the skin it supplies enough medication for pain relief for up to three days. It works by releasing the drug through a permeable membrane and delivers a bolus to the bloodstream through the skin and saturates the subcutaneous fat beneath. Multiple patches may be used to achieve pain relief and they are best used with those people whose pain is already controlled via other routes. It is not effective immediately; therefore other opioids will continue to be given for a few hours. The patch needs to be changed every 72 hours. Side effects are minimal, but skin reactions can occur. One of the most useful side effects is that generally those people stabilised on transdermal fentanyl have fewer constipation problems than those on other major opiates.

- **Rectal** This route is a good alternative when the oral route is not possible due to nausea, vomiting or gastro-intestinal problems. Suppositories are the most suitable form of administration, but any capsule or tablet of any opioid that is used for oral administration can be used rectally (Stevens and Ghazi, 2000). The disadvantages of this route are the delayed or limited absorption of the drug due to the small surface area of the rectum, and constipation or defecation may mean that the drug is absorbed into the faeces instead of the lining of the rectum itself. It can also be very uncomfortable for some patients, and where there are anal fissures, tumours or inflamed haemorrhoids this route should be avoided.

- **Intravenous** This route should really only be considered when other less invasive routes are not appropriate. The advantage is that a bolus can be delivered quickly and effectively to control severe pain in a short time. This then allows the prescription of more appropriate medication via a choice of other routes titrated to the person's needs to stabilize their pain. The disadvantages are principally those associated with an indwelling, central or peripheral catheter, or one-off use of a needle and syringe. Where the skin is broken there is the potential for infection, and skilled care is needed to manage the areas used. Drugs delivered intravenously are also very expensive when compared with oral formulations – a factor which, as we have already stated, is significant in resource-poor environments.

- **Subcutaneous** This is where the drug is injected just below the skin into the subdermal layers. When the oral route is not available this is the simplest and perhaps most reliable route of administration. This route can be used to give medication by bolus (i.e. rapid injection) or continuous slow infusion, and it has a good absorption rate. Skilled care is needed to look after the infusion site, but the rate of skin infections is low (Stevens and Ghazi, 2000). The injection site should be changed weekly or as needed and you should always be alert to skin allergies and the needle displacing into the surrounding tissues.
- **Epidural or intrathecal** This injection-based route is used to place a small dose of an opioid or local anaesthetic close to the spinal receptors situated in the dorsal horn of the spinal cord to enhance analgesia and reduce systemic side effects by decreasing the daily opioid dose (for more information on the dorsal horn, see Chapter 8: *The nature of pain and suffering*). An indwelling catheter is placed in the intrathecal space and the medication is delivered via an external or implantable pump. Complications centre around possible kinking, obstruction or misplacement of the catheter and bleeding at the site of needle insertion.

Although used infrequently these procedures are valuable when complex or intractable pain exists. One advantage is that small doses of opioids are used, and therefore side effects are reduced. Some patients receiving local anaesthetic agents dislike the loss of sensation. Bowel and bladder function can be disturbed. The advice of an anaesthetist, pain or palliative care specialist is essential.

Radiotherapy

Radiotherapy can be very effective to treat the pain caused by bone metastases. The patient may only require one or two treatments and may gain benefit within a few days.

 Reflective activity

For nurses, it is particularly important to be familiar with the different routes for the giving of analgesia and with the drugs available in your place of work. Knowledge of this and your patient, will help you to determine the right analgesic via the right route and to be alert to the possibility of side effects.

Next time you are on duty take a notebook with you and write down the analgesic drugs that are available to you in your work area and the routes of administration. Try looking at the drug charts and the contents of the drug trolley to give yourself an idea. When you have completed your list, log onto palliativedrugs.com, register with the site (this costs you nothing) and access the formulary. Seek out the drugs you have on your list and look at the availability of routes there are for its use. You may well find that there are a number of options available to you that had not been considered before and may be more appropriate for your patients.

Understanding morphine

Morphine is a highly effective and safe analgesic drug. It is widely accepted throughout the world to be the most effective drug of choice for treating cancer pain and other nociceptive pain. The World Health Organization, who endorse this stance, has produced many useful documents to help developing countries understand the nature of morphine and its correct usage for pain relief. This campaign to raise awareness and promote the use of morphine has been highly effective, and currently over 100 countries now have a palliative care strategy which includes the licensing of morphine based drugs for use with chronic cancer pain primarily.

For more information on downloadable documents and books for purchase in this area, log onto the WHO website (http://www.who.int/en/) and type 'pain relief' into their search engine.

It is the responsibility of nurses everywhere to make their colleagues, patients and their families aware of the reality of morphine as a safe and highly effective drug to control pain. It is fair to say that if the prescription of morphine was conducted according to the WHO three-step guidelines where needed, it would transform pain control for hundreds of thousands of people, not only in the UK, but across the world.

Morphine preparations

If at all possible, morphine should be given by mouth. It can be given as immediate release oral morphine solution or as a tablet. Morphine is effective for four hours; therefore it must be given every four hours, **not six or eight hourly**! There is not a standard dose for morphine. It is good practice to administer regular doses of oral morphine every four hours until the correct dose is established. This is known as dose titration.

Remembering to take a pain medication every four hours can be a burden. Morphine is also available in a preparation which is released over twelve hours, for example MST or Zomorph, and there is a 24 hour preparation known as MXL.

There is rarely a place in palliative care for intra-muscular or intravenous injections. Intravenous injections of diamorphine are indicated if a patient has a myocardial infarction or, very occasionally, when severe pain is experienced and control of pain is needed rapidly. Intra-muscular injections are no more effective than subcutaneous injections and they are unpleasant, particularly if the patient has lost a lot of weight.

Diamorphine

Chemically, diamorphine is very similar to morphine, but it has one big advantage over morphine. It is very soluble, therefore it is suitable to be given by injection. Diamorphine may be given by regular subcutaneous injection. Often it is given using a syringe driver. This is a device driven by a battery which slowly and accurately injects medication from a syringe. This method is used when patients are unable to swallow or if they experience troublesome nausea. (For more information about using syringe drivers contact your specialist palliative care nurse or doctor if available.)

Fentanyl

Fentanyl is a powerful opioid analgesic. It is commonly administered intravenously during anaesthesia or in intensive therapy units. It is also available in a 'patch', worn on the skin like a sticking plaster. This method of drug delivery is well established as a method of delivering nicotine in people who wish to stop smoking, and in hormone replacement therapy. Fentanyl delivered by a patch is absorbed slowly through the skin. It is not effective immediately; therefore other opioids will continue to be given for a few hours. The patch needs to be changed every 72 hours. It is useful in patients who have achieved good pain control with other opioids. It is also suggested that patients using the fentanyl patch experience less constipation and are less sleepy during the day than patients taking morphine.

Morphine myths

Unfortunately numerous myths still persist regarding morphine, and the negative press it receives through its misuse as a recreational drug throughout the world has seriously hampered its legitimate licensing and prescription in many countries. Patients, their families and even some health professionals often believe these myths, resulting in poor pain management. It is prudent, therefore, that we take some time to examine these myths and compare them with the facts.

Adverse effects of opioids

These are well known. They are predictable and treatable, and simple, clear explanations will do much to alleviate distress.

- **Constipation**   Almost all patients receiving a mild or strong opioid will become constipated. This will remain an issue for the duration of treatment. Prescribing a regular prophylactic laxative with the opioid can prevent constipation. A combined stimulant and softener is appropriate.
- **Nausea and vomiting**   One to two thirds of patients starting opioids will experience nausea. Within 5–10 days most patients will feel better. They will benefit from prophylactic anti-emetic drugs. Haloperidol or cyclizine are the drugs of choice. Remember that, as well as opioid use, there are many possible causes for nausea in patients with advanced illness.
- **Sedation**   Opioids and other drugs may cause sedation. Patients should be told of this side effect. After a few days it tends to be less of a problem but the dose of drug(s) may need to be altered. The aim is for the person to be alert and pain free.
- **Dry mouth**   Again opioids and other drugs may cause this. Simple remedies such as frequent sips of a favourite drink will help, as will good mouth care.

Less common side effects include hypotension, poor concentration, confusion, urinary hesitancy, itch and respiratory depression.

✎ Reflective activity

Let's see how much you think you know about the reality of morphine usage and its pharmacology.

	TRUE	FALSE
1. Morphine is highly addictive		
2. Morphine will cause respiratory depression		
3. Morphine must not be used too early in an illness to avoid hitting a ceiling dose		

TRUE   FALSE

4. Patients will need more and more morphine as their disease progresses

5. Morphine means this is the end

6. Morphine hastens death

Feedback

Myth	Fact
Morphine is highly addictive	Addiction is a psychological craving for a drug. It is defined only by psychological dependence, i.e. compulsive use of a drug for its mood-altering properties, and continued use despite harm. This is very rare in cancer patients and those with morphine-responsive pain. Patients who 'appear' to be addicted, asking for another dose of medication, are usually still in pain. They 'clock watch' desperate for the next dose to relieve their pain. Patients with a history of drug misuse can still be given opioid analgesics. A pain or palliative care specialist should be consulted for advice.
Morphine will cause respiratory depression	Respiratory depression is very rare in the person whose opioid dose has been carefully titrated to their pain. Indeed, pain itself is a strong respiratory stimulant. Study has shown that in a group of terminally ill patients with respiratory failure and dyspnoea, administration of subcutaneous morphine improved dyspnoea without causing significant deterioration in respiratory function. *If* respiratory depression occurs it can be managed with a drug called naloxone.
Morphine must not be used too early in an illness to avoid hitting a ceiling dose	There is no ceiling to the prescription of morphine where it is used for nociceptive pain. As the dose is raised the analgesic effects increase.
Patients will need more and more morphine as their disease progresses	This is not usual. If patients do require escalating doses it is often a sign that the pain is not responding well to morphine, or that other drugs or interventions are more appropriate.
Morphine means this is the end	Sadly many patients believe this. It is understandable because most of the information they have received during their lives will have been negative. Some professionals also believe this and withhold morphine until the patient is near the end of life. At times, nurses blame doctors for not prescribing sufficient morphine. This may be true, but nurses sometimes withhold medication that has been prescribed correctly, believing it to be harmful.
Morphine hastens death	Despite media hype there is no real evidence that morphine doses, carefully titrated to the patient, hasten death. A major study conducted by Berkovitch *et al.* (1999) found that 'high morphine dosage does not affect patient survival'.

Titrating and converting drug dosages

Whilst the prescription of controlled drugs is primarily a medical province, it is essential that nurses know how to initiate, maintain and convert dosages so that they can be in a position both to observe correct practice and to advise when the medical staff are inexperienced and may shy away from prescribing appropriate pain relief.

Opioids should be used for control of pain as indicated in the WHO analgesic ladder. The opioid dose required to control an individual's pain will depend on many factors and is not related to any one parameter. The correct titration of dose is the key to success and will minimise the risk of either overdose or unwanted side effects.

Normal release morphine preparations have an onset of action of about 20 minutes and reach peak drug levels on average at 60 minutes. The rapid onset of analgesia makes these preparations more suitable for use in initiating therapy for severe pain and for treating breakthrough pain. Usually normal release preparations must be given every four hours to maintain a constant analgesic level and when given in this way these preparations will reach a steady plasma concentration and hence full effect within 12–15 hours.

This means that the full effect of any dose change can be assessed at this time. In practice, during titration dose adjustments are usually made every 24 hours unless the pain is more severe when adjustments may be made sooner.

Controlled release morphine preparations have a slower onset and later peak effect. Many of the twice daily preparations have an onset of action of 1–2 hours and reach peak drug levels at 4 hours. The once daily preparations have a slower onset and reach peak drug levels at 8.5 hours. This means that controlled release preparations generally do not allow rapid titration for patients in severe pain, due to slow onset and the long dosing intervals.

With this in mind, titration should therefore be carried out with a normal release morphine preparation given every four hours to maintain constant analgesic levels. At bed time, however, it is useful to give double the dose; then the night time dose is unlikely to be required. When good pain relief has been achieved it is appropriate to convert to controlled/sustained release preparations if available.

Much confusion and worry exists about how and when to do this conversion without compromising the patient's pain relief. The principles are straightforward and if followed correctly a successful transition is usually achieved.

Always remember that 3 mg of oral morphine = 1 mg SC diamorphine, so the approximate relative potencies of oral morphine and subcutaneous diamorphine are:

Oral morphine (mg/24 h)	90	180	240
Subcutaneous diamorphine (mg/24 h)	30	60	80

These are the approximate relative potencies of oral morphine, transdermal fentanyl and subcutaneous diamorphine:

4 hourly oral morphine (mg)	24 hourly oral morphine (mg)	Fentanyl patch (mcg/h)	24 hourly SC Diamorphine (mg)
5–20	30–120	25	10–40
25–35	140–220	50	50–70
40–50	230–310	75	80–100
55–65	320–400	100	110–130

The doses advised in this table are approximations for guidance only and should always be titrated to the individual patient's requirements. When pain is controlled, add up the total daily dose of normal release morphine the patient is receiving and give this equivalent dose as a once daily controlled release preparation, or divide the 24 hour total dose by two and give this dose as a twice daily controlled release preparation.

Remember also, when transferring a patient from four hourly normal release morphine to a controlled release preparation, to start the controlled release preparation at the time the next normal release morphine dose is due, and discontinue the regular normal release morphine from this time onwards. Figure 10.2 is a useful diagram which outlines the progression of dosage prescription, titration and the correct pathway to follow.

Current recommendations based on the best research evidence available produced for the European Association for Palliative Care (Hanks *et al.*, 2001) and endorsed by the WHO are to start with a prescription of 10 mg of oral morphine every 4 hours (unless the patient has known renal problems) and a breakthrough dose of 10 mg if necessary. The amount of morphine given over the first 24 hours needs to be monitored carefully and the pain reassessed after 24 hours with the dosage adjusted according to the efficacy of the regime. If the dosage needs to be increased then increments of between 25 and 50% are usual.

So a dose of 10 mg × 4 hourly = 60 mg over 24 hours. Increasing the dose to 90 mg over 24 hours would be appropriate, for instance 15 mg × 4 hourly. A double dose of oral morphine, for example 20 mg, at night time is an effective and safe way of ensuring a good night's sleep.

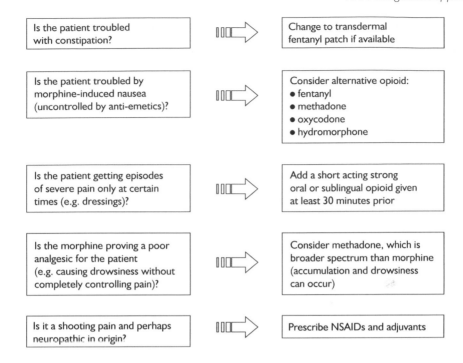

Figure 10.2 The progression of dosage prescription and titration.

Breakthrough pain

Regular doses of appropriate analgesia successfully titrated manages pain in the vast majority of patients. Pain, however, may return between regular doses, particularly if the patient is very active or the disease has rapidly progressed. This is called 'breakthrough pain'. When breakthrough pain like this occurs the aim is to provide the patient with a supplementary dose of opioids to get on top of that pain quickly and effectively.

The characteristics of such pain are usually rapid onset, moderate to severe in intensity with the pain being of relatively short duration, for example 15–30 minutes. Episodes often occur up to four times daily and can seriously interfere with the patient's quality of life.

Managing this pain is straightforward as long as those prescribing the medication follow a very simple formula (EAPC, 1996):

1. Calculate total daily (24 hour) dose of the oral medication prescribed (for example 120 mg sustained-release morphine).
2. Use 1/6th of this amount for the breakthrough pain dosage (for example 20 mg immediate-release morphine).

Or another example:

1. A patient receiving 40 mg of oral immediate release morphine every four hours will have a total 24 hour dose of 240 mg (40 × 6 = 240).
2. The breakthrough dose prescribed at 1/6th should therefore be 40 mg.

Factors such as a full stomach or decreased gastric emptying time, may delay the absorption rates and the speed of onset of any analgesics administered orally and this should be borne in mind.

There may be occasions when a painful procedure needs to be performed, and in this case additional doses of analgesic drugs should be given well beforehand so that breakthrough pain does not happen. Anticipating such events is all part of good nursing practice and nurses should be sure that an intervention is really necessary before carrying it out.

Following the delivery of oral breakthrough analgesia wait 30 minutes to assess the response. If the pain persists then repeat the analgesia and reassess in a further 30 minutes. If pain still persists a full reassessment of the patient's pain is required. Because of the anxiety generated by such pain it is important that there is a careful explanation of the correct use of breakthrough analgesia to both the patient and their carers if appropriate.

 Reflective activity

Using the 1/6th of the 24 hour dosage principle, check out the prescription of analgesics in your work area and practice working out the correct breakthrough pain prescription for these dosages. Also check against the prescription chart to see if such a dose has been included in the regime.

What are adjuvant drugs?

Although not thought of as analgesic drugs, other drugs can be used to manage pain in patients with advanced illness. These agents do not necessarily treat the pain itself, but can be used in combination with major opiates to increase or aid their effectiveness. You should always check with your local specialist palliative care services if unsure about which drug to use and in what dosage or combination.

- **Antidepressants**: amitriptyline can be used to manage neuropathic pain. Given in small doses amitriptyline is not used to manage depression. It works by modifying the transmission of pain impulses.

- **Anticonvulsants**: carbamazepine, sodium valproate and gabapentin also modify pain impulses.
- **Antispamodics**: hyoscine butylbromide and hyoscine hydrobromide relieve pain by reducing smooth muscle contraction. Particularly helpful in bowel colic.
- **Antispastics**: are helpful in skeletal muscle tension in multiple sclerosis. Diazepam and other medications have been used to good effect.
- **Corticosteroids**: cortisone, prednisolone and dexamethasone work by reducing inflammation surrounding tumours.
- **Antibiotics**: are highly effective in reducing pain due to inflammation when the cause is infection.
- **Muscle relaxants**: for painful muscle spasm (cramp) and myofascial pain, the correct approach is local heat, massage in the first instance, but also benzodiazepine, diazepam and relaxation therapy can be useful.
- **Bisphosphonates**: These are osteoclast inhibitors and are used to relieve metastatic bone pain which persists despite analgesics and radiotherapy surgery.
- **Neuropathic agents**: Drugs in this category are most commonly used when neuropathic pain does not respond well to standard analgesics together with an antidepressant and an anti-epileptic. They have also been used in inflammatory pain, for example severe mucositis. Drugs available include: ketamine, methadone and amantadine.

Non-pharmacological approaches to pain management

There are a wide range of strategies and treatments that are available to you to utilise in the management of pain without using invasive pharmacology. As you will see, many are simple and inexpensive, whilst others may require more careful thinking. All are a challenge to nursing practice, but are proven to work in multiple environments.

The simple quality of life options

It is always useful to start with those strategies and activities that are sometimes forgotten in the quest for successful pain relief. As we have seen so far, managing pain is an art and a science and getting the balance right is not always easy. Consider the options below for example:

- The help, advice and support of another professional such as a physiotherapist, occupational therapist, psychologist or social worker
- Heat or cold
- A soak in a deep warm bath
- Someone to talk to
- Someone who will listen but not judge when the patient is sad, angry or confused
- Distraction, for example watching television or reading a book
- A gentle massage
- A comfortable bed and chair
- A good night's sleep
- Good food and company

Think about what you can do to facilitate the above. You may think you don't have the skills to provide some of the comfort measures suggested above. It is not necessary to attend a massage course to give a hand massage, although you should not use aromatherapy products without permission. Massage and other comfort measures show that you have time for the patient and put you in a place where you have time to listen and respond to the patient's worries and concerns. This, in itself, may help to reduce pain.

 Reflective activity

Take a look down the bullet list above and ask yourself which of these you utilise already in your personal life to relieve emotional, spiritual and/or physical pain. Make a note of the most successful ones and what it was about those activities that worked for you.

What else can be done to manage pain?

Analgesic drugs will always form the foundation of pain management in advanced illness, but there are a number of other pain relieving approaches that a nurse can exploit as part of their role.

- **Trans-cutaneous electrical nerve stimulation (TENS)**
  This device has been used for many years to help in the management of different types of pain. It has proved useful in pain due to trapped nerves like in sciatica and for people who get phantom limb pain after an amputation. The TENS equipment consists of three parts, the stimulator, the leads and the electrodes. The stimulator is powered by a 9 volt battery. The electrodes

are made of carbon rubber. They are placed, usually, near the pain and the stimulator is adjusted to create a feeling of gentle but strong stimulation in the skin. Sometimes pain relief is immediate, while in some people it may take time to be effective. With TENS the patient is in control. TENS will not be effective in all types of pain, but may be a useful addition to other approaches. Patients may be referred to a pain clinic for specialist advice.

■ **Relaxation**

Pain causes muscle tension and tense muscles ache, causing more pain. Teaching simple relaxation exercises helps the patient to bring muscle tension under control and break the cycle. Relaxation and imagery are part of a range of techniques which can bring comfort to the dying and bereaved. Benefits of relaxation include:

– Reduction in autonomic activity
– Lower pulse
– Lower blood pressure
– Lower temperature
– Decreased muscular tension
– Pain reduction
– Aids rest and sleep
– Feeling of wellbeing
– Feeling of control and mastery

Relaxation methods aim to reduce tension by physical, psychological, spiritual or combined approaches. Like all skills, relaxation requires practice to become proficient. Ideally, patients would learn to relax in a quiet warm environment free of interruptions. These conditions are difficult to attain in real life, yet patients say they can learn to relax in the most challenging situations.

■ **Progressive muscular relaxation**

This is the easiest method to teach and to learn. The patient is guided through a sequence of simple and straightforward tensing and relaxing exercises so that he or she can become aware of the difference between tension and relaxation. It can begin with the patient tensing and relaxing hands and arms and then working from head to toe. It is important to know the patient in terms of their pain so that painful areas can be avoided.

■ **Guided imagery or fantasy**

Relaxing images are used to help patients divert attention from where they are to an imaginary scene, such as a favourite holiday scene or a comforting image of home. The teacher can use his or her own images or make use of the patient's own images. Occasionally patients find they are unable to see an image in their 'mind's eye'.

■ **Autogenic relaxation**

This method consists of a series of easy mental exercises designed to switch off the 'fight or flight' response in the body and replace it with a relaxation response. Autogenic relaxation is usually taught in a group over a series of weeks. Training consists of learning basic exercises which involve visualising particular instructions such as feelings of heaviness, warmth and coolness in different parts of the body. It is claimed to be helpful in stress-related disorders. In palliative care it can be adapted and taught in shorter sessions.

- **Hypnosis/hypnotherapy**
  The general public and some healthcare professionals sometimes think of hypnosis as something mystical and magical. Hypnotherapy aims to facilitate an altered state of consciousness in which the mind becomes very deeply relaxed. In such a state the patient is very susceptible to positive and beneficial suggestions. It has been used in palliative care, where it has many practical applications (e.g. pain management, management of symptoms such as nausea and vomiting, particularly anticipatory vomiting and dyspnoea, fear and anxiety management and phobia management). Hypnotherapy is a safe and effective approach but should only be used by those who have been specifically trained.

- **Meditation**
  Meditation is another approach to relaxation that requires the user to practice quiet relaxation. A mantra is used as a focus to deepen the relaxation. The mantra is usually a neutral sound without specific meaning which is repeated silently over and over again. This helps the user to concentrate thoughts inwardly and almost block out the outside world. Concentrating on objects such as a candle in a darkened room, or a flower or pleasant odours, is a useful alternative to the mantra. The patient with advanced illness is unlikely to be able to devote extended periods of time to meditation. Nevertheless, many patients may be able to deepen their relaxation by applying the principles of meditation.

- **Deep breathing**
  Teachers often ask their subjects to focus on their breathing, or become aware of and notice their breathing. This is undoubtedly helpful for some patients, but unhelpful for others. Approximately 50% of patients with advanced cancer have difficulty in breathing. Focusing on breathing may be helpful, but conversely may cause distress. If in doubt it may be better to avoid mentioning breathing.

You may have learned relaxation skills on placements such as maternity or mental health. After consulting with your qualified colleagues, consider their use in patients with advanced illness. Combine relaxation, where possible, with nursing measures such as bathing, wound care or when you notice a patient appears tense.

Other relaxation strategies include:

- **Talking/chatting** – Normal conversation about daily life can be very helpful at distracting the patient away from troubling issues.
- **Family support** – The family are often physically and mentally exhausted so need to be looked after and their contribution to caring valued openly by the healthcare team.
- **Counselling** – Not always appropriate, but in circumstances where it is clear there are deep seated issues that the person wishes to resolve, this can be helpful.
- **Befriending** – Do not underestimate the value of your presence and the trusted relationship you may have with the person. This can be a powerful aid to easing the suffering of a person.
- **Reminiscence** – Helping the person to review significant events in their life has been shown to help give meaning to people about their suffering and has the potential to facilitate changes in attitude and behaviour.
- **Life story books** – This is a strategy that has been used effectively for many years by parents who have lost or are about to lose a child and by children who have lost or are about to lose a parent. It involves collecting together pictures and mementos and putting them into a book that chronicles the person's life. It can be just as helpful adult to adult.
- **Cognitive and behavioural therapies** – These talking therapies are designed to be used in a structured, formalised setting with trained and experienced therapists. They have the potential to help people change difficult behaviour and thought patterns that seriously impede quality of life.
- **Massage** – One of the simplest and most therapeutic forms of touch a nurse can ever use with a patient. It is not necessary to attend a course or be formally qualified to use gentle massage on the hands and feet as long as simple safety precautions are observed. Establish that this is acceptable to the patient: some cultures may find it offensive and there may be gender issues. Talk to the patient where possible to establish that there are no open cuts, or abrasions, and no arthritic or swollen joints. If there are any other lesions or tumours visible, then massage is clearly contraindicated. Find out what is available and what the patient prefers in terms of hand creams, or perhaps aromatherapy oils.
- **Wound care** – Dressings that are secure and free from leakage can help patient comfort enormously. Remember to instigate a regular assessment of the wound's condition. If the wound is causing direct pain then consider appropriate analgesia.
- **Visits** – If the person is being cared for in an institutional environment then no matter how friendly the staff they will miss the support of family and friends, which can have a knock-on effect for their pain relief. Find out from the patient who is important in their life and do not always assume that it is immediate family. Be aware that the patient may tire easily with too many people around and be their advocate when necessary to limit time spent at the bedside. Find out what the visiting policy is and remember

issues such as parking, refreshments and chairs around the bed. Consider open visiting if the family has to travel a long distance. The key element is to remain discreetly in the background, but available.

- **Diet/nutrition** – There is clear evidence that cachexia from both the disease process and aggravated by poor nutrition can impede physiological well-being and pain management. The key things to remember here are small meals, high in calories to boost energy, that are well presented. Assessment of nutritional likes and dislikes should be made and meals should be modified to suit the person's wishes. If feeding is needed then time should be allowed for this important and often neglected function.

- **Entertainment** – Ill people who may be in pain can have poor concentration, but it is still important to consider carefully how the person can fill their day. What is available to you will depend on your situation, and newspapers, magazines, books, TV with remote control, CD and radios, walkmans, headphones (with plenty of batteries) are all activities which can provide a little relief and occupy a patient's mind. Diversional therapy, such as card making, knitting, painting, jigsaw puzzles and games, can be very helpful. All have their place to distract the person from their pain experience and may even provide some spiritual support.

- **Sleep and rest** – Often forgotten, but vital to the successful relief of debilitating pain. Make sure that there are quiet periods for the patient and reduce intrusive noise where possible (e.g. TV, radio, medication trolleys). Consider alternatives to sleep-inducing agents, such as milky drinks, small amounts of alcohol, relaxing music and ear plugs.

- **Spiritual issues** – Where a person has a personal faith that guides their life it is usually possible to find a representative of that faith who can offer support in terms of the rituals and practices that go with that religion. Suffering is multidimensional, as we know, and much relief can be obtained through the strength and solace of a personal faith. Not everyone has a faith, however, yet the need for spiritual support can be given in other ways. Time alone and with those who matter, peace, quiet and solitude can all help give meaning to the pain experience. Do not forget also the important aesthetic beauty that enhances life quality for all humanity, for example nature, sunrise and sunset, chocolate and music.

- **Acupuncture/pressure** – This active treatment has a long tradition for its efficacy in managing certain types of pain and has been in use in far-eastern cultures for over 2,000 years. Expertise in this area in western cultures is increasing all the time and where carefully selected and used it can help in pain relief.

Reflective activity

Look again at the concept of 'total pain' and ask yourself to what extent are you utilising the art as well as the science of pain management in your work environment? Make a note of the activities that take place in your work area to manage pain beyond the prescription of drugs.

If your list is small then think back to a time when you were in pain. Apart from taking pain medications, what did you do to ease the pain? What made things worse? What made things better? What helped when you were a child?

Feedback: Hopefully you will have scanned through the extensive list of options and selected those that are realistic and achievable in your current work environment. Not all are appropriate for all people, and the influence of culture, religious practice, material resources and local policies will have a bearing on what you can achieve.

If you had difficulty with this activity maybe it's because you are still thinking in terms of pain as a *physical* entity only and not as the 'total' pain experience for the patient. This takes practice and its challenge should not be underestimated.

Formulating your pain management strategy

Now that you have reached this point you are ready to begin to put your knowledge together and to formulate a workable strategy that you can take into your work area. If you have been engaging with the reflective activities so far you will already have looked at your current practice and challenged your thinking about what could be done to improve pain relief.

Perhaps one of the simplest methods of remembering a strategy is to use the 'step' approach, just as the WHO did so successfully with the analgesic ladder. The following approach is offered to you as just one way of organising your thinking to address the patient's needs.

Each person will need an individual plan depending on the cause, site, and nature of their pain or pains.

Step 1 – Use your good listening and attending skills to facilitate a conversation with the person so that you can explain the cause of the pain.
Step 2 – Tell the person what the treatment options are for their pain.
Step 3 – Think holistically and begin your regime.
Step 4 – Add in other therapeutic options as appropriate.
Step 5 – Review and review again.

Or to put it even more simply – Talk – Do – Review.

Reflective activity

See if you can work out a simple mnemonic to help you remember the sequence of events. A mnemonic is an arrangement of letters to form either a real or made-up word or rhyme that can help you remember a sequence. For example, here is one that can be used for pain assessment:

SOCRATES
Site
Onset
Character
Radiation
Alleviating factors/**A**ssociated symptoms
Timing (duration, frequency)
Exacerbating factors
Severity

Feedback: You may have come up with a simple made-up word like:

COBAR
Cause
Options
Begin
Add
Review

Applying pain management strategies to a case study

Read the background information through carefully and then the assessment of Judith's pain that was described in Chapter 9: *The assessment of pain*. This should give you a good idea about what to do next.

Reviewing the assessment of pain

This is the background information to the case study which you will need to read in order to place in context the assessment of Judith's pain and which will influence your proposed management strategy.

This married couple are both 46 years old and live in a small housing estate on the edge of town. John is a labourer and is often out of work, whilst Judith has a part time job at a local clothing factory. Their son Christopher (9) is a bright but quiet lad who is very close to his father. John and his son share a love of fishing and spend most weekends at the local lake. The family are practising Christians. Judith was married before to Tom, who lives nearby with their two teenage children from this marriage (Henry, 12, and Nikki, 14) and his new wife. They all get on reasonably well, but the two elder children sometimes behave badly towards Christopher.

They are a close, trusting and caring family who have few friends and lead a very private life. Judith has an old school friend called Cheryl who is a trusted confidante, living a few doors away, but John is very much a loner. He is the main decision maker, who sees himself as the traditional head of the family, and Judith has a rather nervous disposition and is inclined to panic at times over relatively minor things. Judith's elderly mother died six months ago after a long illness. She lived a long way from their home and Judith could not provide the support she wanted for her because of the distance. John's family emigrated many years prior and he has no contact with them.

Recently Judith has been feeling unwell and has not been eating properly. She has had a lot of indigestion and heartburn and eventually went to her family doctor. He sent her for investigations and an epigastric mass was found. The consultant decided to get her into hospital as soon as possible for an exploratory laparotomy. A huge gastric tumour was found with extensive liver and pelvic deposits with bone involvement. The surgeons closed her up with no procedure done.

You will notice that this family are essentially based in a western society, have Christian beliefs and values and have access to a well organised model of healthcare. Whilst this may not be representative of many countries, they are nevertheless traditional in their structure and thinking, working class in their income and, as you will see, have mostly the same issues and concerns that any family would have worldwide.

Judith's pain

Judith was given some Pethidine post-operatively which was successful in controlling her pain over the first 12–24 hours. It is now five days since the surgery and she continues to be nauseous throughout the day. Her abdominal pain, however, is steadily getting worse and is radiating down her back. It is constant and she can only get some comfort by curling into the foetal position, which she maintains for hours at a time. Her mood is now low and she communicates little to the staff. She is uncomplaining of pain, but her facial expressions, mannerisms and behaviour suggest otherwise. The night staff say that she is crying a lot in the early hours. The hospital chaplain has been to see her, as has her parish vicar. She seems to get some comfort from their visits, but voices are sometimes raised in anger and they leave soon after.

She has also started complaining of headaches and gastritis, which seem to get worse before and after she has a visit from her family or the doctor. She wants to go home as soon as possible, but is concerned about whether her family will be able to cope and tries hard to convince the team that her pain is much better and she will be okay.

Judith's pain assessment

In the interview with Judith much time was spent trying to convince you that she is not suffering much pain and is able to go home. However, here we have a situation where the McCaffery (1972) definition of pain, 'pain is what the experiencing person says it is, existing whenever he says it does' could be challenged. Judith's priority to go home has to be balanced against her answers to your questions and your and the team's observations of Judith's body language and behaviour throughout the day, coupled with any information her family may be able to supply you. Note that two out of three of her pains are *not* caused by her cancer.

Using the framework for the pain assessment interview suggested in Chapter 9, this is a précised version of the result that was achieved.

- **Look and listen**: The main issues for Judith centre around getting herself well enough to go home to her family for the last period of her life. Her conversation is dominated by this, so it's important to listen carefully and acknowledge the reality of her pain experience.
- **Consider the person's age, cultural background and ability to respond**: Judith is still a young woman at 46 and is having to face the prospect of not seeing any of her children grow up, as well as not fulfilling a long relationship with her husband. Although she is a private lady she is also known to be an anxious person. Trust is important for someone like her and your skills at developing a rapport with her will help you to get some honest replies regarding her pain. She has a strong personal faith which may give her immense spiritual support or be severely challenged by this illness.
- **Listen actively to the problems in the patient's order of priority**: Her quality of life issues may be very different from how you perceive them regarding her pain. In this case Judith is trying to hide the severity of her pain so that she can get home as soon as possible.

- **Think of possible causes**: As your interview progresses with Judith you begin to get a better picture of the holistic nature of her pain, and causes may well spring to mind quite quickly. As well as the more obvious physical pains, don't forget the psychosocial element, for example:
  - Fear of losing control over her life and independence
  - Worries over her son Christopher and his future and the difficult relationship with Henry and Nikki, who may feel shut out
  - Anxiety regarding the home and financial security
- **Use assessment tools to help**: The numerical, verbal and pictorial pain scales are all appropriate to use with Judith in your assessment. It may also be useful for the staff to keep a diary of her pain over 24 hours. Normally it would be Judith who would keep a diary, but bearing in mind her behaviour and her goal to go home as soon as possible, she is likely not to be honest in her reporting. Judith's scores on the numerical and pictorial scales are in the middle range consistently, despite her grimacing and body language, which imply much stronger pain.
- **Explore options**: This is the key part of the management of her pain and will be covered in detail in the next unit of study.
- **Plan**: Once Judith, her family and the team have agreed the way forward, the management can begin. Clear and up-to-date documentation of your assessment of her pain and the subsequent management strategy is vital. Make sure that all the relevant team members are aware.
- **Explain**: Judith's husband will almost certainly want to know the outcome of your assessment. It is normally good practice to ask Judith's permission first before telling him, but this depends on the cultural norms within your healthcare system.
- **Review**: If the management strategy is effective then Judith's pain will alter radically over the next 24 hours. In the first instance it would be appropriate to review her pain after 1–2 hours and 6 hourly thereafter. After 24 hours it will depend on the resources you have available, i.e. drug availability and support systems, but ideally it should be done once a day until her pain is well controlled.

✐ Reflective activity:

Put together a pain relief regime that you think will help to control Judith's pain. Use the structure suggested to you above. Use your knowledge of pain management approaches, Judith's assessment and overall condition to put the regime together. Consider the short- and long-term issues to enable her to go home to her family as she wishes.

Feedback: Judith's suggested pain management regime:

Step 1 – Talk: It is quite clear that Judith has three separate pains of different origin and that each will necessitate a different approach. Her psychological, spiritual and social needs also impact on the regime significantly.

■ Her gastritis and headaches would seem to be related to her anxiety and visits from the priest and her family, therefore may well be psychosomatic in origin. This does not mean that we should ignore them, but for the moment they are not the priority.
■ Her abdominal pain that is radiating down her back is without doubt the main priority and in the first instance it would be good practice to give her a stat (once only) dose of diamorphine 5–10 mg by injection to give her some rapid relief from this crippling pain. It may also be appropriate to give her an anxiolytic such as diazepam 5–10 mg to relax her and help relieve the anxiety she is experiencing.
■ This should take effect within 5–10 minutes and will enable you then to sit by her side and talk through the treatment options with her knowing that she will be better able to concentrate on what you have to say. The rapid effect of the diamorphine will also boost her confidence in your approach and she is likely to be more willing to comply with a suitable regime than previously.

Step 2 – Tell: Her pain is not now related to the post-operative period (pethidine was the right choice at the time, but is only effective for short time spans and as such is not useful chronic pain relief). It is likely that the pain is directly related to her cancer and will therefore most likely be nociceptive in origin and opiate responsive. It is unlikely that Step One of the ladder will be effective for her, considering her pain history and body language, so ask yourself whether it is appropriate to go to Step Two or Three of the analgesic ladder. Her pain could not really be described as moderate despite the scores on the pain scales in her assessment.

Using the guidance from the WHO given in Module 2 Unit 3, Judith can be prescribed a starting dose of 10 mg oral morphine every 4 hours for the first 24 hours, after which the pain needs to be reassessed. A PRN (as necessary) dose of 10 mg of oral morphine needs to be prescribed alongside in case of breakthrough pain and the amount given over the first 24 hours monitored closely.

An appropriate laxative will also need to be prescribed, e.g. Codanthrusate. Lastly a prescription of an appropriate oral antacid for her gastritis, to be given as necessary, would be useful. All this will need to be explained carefully to Judith so that she and her husband understand the nature of the drug regime and how it works.

Don't forget to think holistically. A quiet warm room or bay, as she prefers, may be a good option if available and spending time with her, even when procedures are complete, will help ease her anxiety and support the whole family. As morphine can cause a dry mouth there will be a need to monitor her oral hygiene and promote drinks of high calories both to hydrate her and to offset any potential cachexia in the longer term.

It is also important to assess her risk of pressure sores and to use appropriate aids where available alongside close monitoring of her skin by the nursing staff.

Step 3 – Begin: If the pain is well controlled then Judith needs to be monitored closely for the next few days and her regime stabilised. If it is not well controlled and needs adjusting upwards then upping the overall 24 hour dose by 50% is acceptable, i.e. from 60 mg to 90 mg (10 mg to 15 mg × 4 hourly).

Find out what she likes to do in the day and use massage of hands or feet, aromatherapy oils, and quiet music to create a calm and therapeutic ambience. She may like to read or watch TV or receive more visitors. Always ask her permission regarding visitors, as she may become tired very quickly if they overstay their visit.

Step 4 – Add: Be aware that about 20% of cancer pain may not respond to opiates; therefore a range of adjuvant drugs such as gabapentin or amitriptyline for neuropathic pain may need to be prescribed to control her pain. This will depend entirely on her response to the regime and the type of pain she is experiencing.

Although she is not complaining of nausea, a significant proportion of those prescribed opiates will experience this at some time, so an 'as necessary' prescription of an anti-emetic, for example cyclizine or haloperidol, may be appropriate.

It is likely that her headache is anxiety related, so once her cancer pain and other issues have been addressed then it may well disappear. If it does not, then an anti-inflammatory analgesic such as ibuprofen can be effective. Headaches do not respond well to morphine so a different approach is needed.

Don't forget that she has a personal faith, so ask her about how she would like to receive spiritual support in this difficult time. Do not assume that she wants a church minister. It may be that she has a network of friends from within her faith community who could help, or even a supportive conversation with those nurses and staff she likes and trusts. Spiritual care takes many forms and is a very individual concept.

Step 5 – Review: It is quite possible that her pain may be bony in origin, therefore palliative radiotherapy to that specific area may be a relevant choice. The benefits and effects of this will need to be carefully explained to Judith. If a syringe driver is available then keep this as a last resort only if she begins to vomit regularly. Remember the golden rules   by the mouth, by the clock and by the ladder.

In the longer term her pain management regime will need to be reviewed so that she can be stabilised on controlled release oral or patch medication (e.g. MXL or norcap or fentanyl patches). This will be much easier for her to manage and will enhance her quality of life hugely. She will, of course need to have appropriate prescriptions for constipation and any other side effects she may be experiencing.

Achieving a successful regime is always a balancing act between keeping the person pain-free and reducing the associated side effects and symptoms. The best judge of your success will be Judith herself and her family. Your aim is to improve her quality of life in all its dimensions by addressing the whole person via the 'total' pain approach.

Competency in pain management

This section concerns itself with your ability to manage pain in your work environment using the facilities available to you. It is recognised that care takes place in many varied circumstances and few are ideal, but the competency assessment offered to you here is intended to allow you to apply the learning you have achieved so far in this chapter and to review and reflect on the reality of what can be achieved, and indeed what you have already achieved.

The skills required to manage pain

Just how competent are you to manage pain and how do you know that the skills you have developed are based around a sound evidence base? Work by people like Benner (1984), who writes about nurses moving from 'novice to expert' on a continuum, provides us with a clear idea of the ways in which adults learn in the 'real world' of practice.

If you have attempted the activities in this chapter and the previous chapters on the nature of pain and the assessment of pain you will already have a good level of knowledge. Such activities are useful to consolidate learning and this kind of reflective process is very useful, but the ability to think and write effectively does not necessarily translate into competence in clinical skills. This is why it is important that we take an honest and critical look at our perceived level of skills in pain management so that we can work towards improving our practice.

What is a competency?

There are numerous definitions available for the term *competency*, but for our purposes we will concentrate on the definition cited by the RCN (2002, p. 2) in relation to specialist palliative nursing. Competence in a given set of skills can be defined as 'The skills, knowledge, experience, attributes and behaviours required by an individual in order to perform the job effectively'. In order to work, therefore, it relies on the formulation of agreed competency statements that are then identified at differing levels of practice.

What is the graduated scale used?

- **Explored**: To examine and investigate systematically an area or skill related to practice.
- **Practised**: To take a skill and use it appropriately in the clinical area on a repeated basis.
- **Developed**: To progress in the knowledge, application and evaluation of a skill and demonstrate this in practice.

This scale has been taken from the generic assessment tool in palliative nursing devised by Becker (2000).

What do I do?

1. Read the competency statements (p. 208) thoroughly and familiarise your-self with the grading structure.
2. Set some time aside to conduct your own self-assessment of your current skills level. This will help you to identify areas for development, which can be addressed in your clinical practice.
3. It is helpful if you can select perhaps 2–3 competencies that are priorities and these may be written into a learning contract (p. 209) to help you focus on what needs to be done to move your skills forward (a suggested format for a learning contract is offered to you). The real learning and development rests upon your ability to examine the deficits, and plan a strategy to deal with these issues in your everyday practice.

This process has the added advantage of clarifying and validating for you what you perceive you are competent at and where this is evident. This is important for our professional development, as sometimes it can be difficult to acknowledge and articulate what we know we are good at in our job when the culture of nursing is so often centred on identifying the problems rather than the achievements.

The success of this approach lies in your ability to be both honest and reflective in your assessment. It is undoubtedly challenging both intellectually and personally to put one's perceived skills so closely under scrutiny, but if we are to improve the care of those in pain then it is important to define clearly what it is we expect a nurse to do, and what should be the standard of care. The evidence base presented by this competency process is but one small step in this direction and is offered to you as an opportunity to engage in such work.

Pain management competencies

	Explored	Practised	Developed
1. Demonstrate and articulate an active commitment to the relief of pain and the palliation of distressing symptoms			
2. Apply knowledge of the nature of pain and assessment of pain to the clinical management of pain			
3. Demonstrate a sound knowledge of the WHO analgesic ladder and discuss the appropriate use of opiates and adjuvant therapies			
4. Explore the concepts of autonomy and compliance relating to pain management			
5. Describe the means by which oral opiate doses are calculated for administration			
6. Organise and initiate the administration of appropriate pain medication, regularly reviewing the situation, anticipating possible problems and reacting to presenting problems			
7. Advise the patient and family where appropriate and acceptable, on the range of possible options to help alleviate pain			
8. Recognise situations where a range of alternative strategies and psychological and spiritual support can benefit the patient in the management and control of total pain			
9. Regularly review pain management to enable an effective pain management strategy			
10. Demonstrate competency in the management of total pain			

Consolidating your learning

Now that you have actively taken the time to examine your skills level and hopefully worked on a strategy to improve your pain management skills, this will help you consolidate your learning.

It can be helpful to revisit your original assessment and to rescore yourself after a period of time (p. 210). (It is suggested that you may need a week or two to do this, but it is entirely dependent on your individual circumstances.)

Suggested learning contract

Identified pain assessment competency:

Self-assessment rating:
Explored ☐   **Practised** ☐   **Developed** ☐

Resources and Strategies (What do I need to do to improve my competency level?)

Evidence of Accomplishment (How can I demonstrate what I have learnt?)

Target Date: ....

Criteria for validating skills accomplishment:

How do you now judge your skill in this competency?

Explored ☐   **Practised** ☐   **Developed** ☐

	Your original score			Your score now		
	Explored	Practised	Developed	Explored	Practised	Developed
1. Demonstrate and articulate an active commitment to the relief of pain and the palliation of distressing symptoms						
2. Apply knowledge of the nature of pain and assessment of pain to the clinical management of pain						
3. Demonstrate a sound knowledge of the WHO analgesic ladder and discuss the appropriate use of opiates and adjuvant therapies						
4. Explore the concepts of autonomy and compliance relating to pain management						
5. Describe the means by which oral opiate doses are calculated for administration						
6. Organise and initiate the administration of appropriate pain medication, regularly reviewing the situation, anticipating problems and reacting to presenting problems						
7. Advise the patient and family where appropriate on the range of possible options to help alleviate pain						
8. Recognise situations where a range of alternative strategies and psychological and spiritual support can benefit the patient in the management and control of total pain						
9. Regularly review pain management to enable an effective pain management strategy						
10. Demonstrate competency in the management of total pain						

Reflective activity

Try to answer the next few questions and keep a note of your responses.

- Some of your scores may have moved right across the scale and others not moved at all. Write down a few notes as to why this is so. What helped or hindered you in your attempts to improve your pain management skills?
- In an exercise like this there are nearly always things that you have done that on reflection you would have done differently. Write down what these are and what it is you will do differently next time.
- What insights have you gained about your own skills in pain management? For example:
  - Were you surprised at how good you were?
  - Were you surprised at how bad you were?
  - Did you expose your knowledge limitations and feel awkward at times?
  - Did you find out things about your patients that surprised you?
  - Did it confirm what you already knew?
- This is the difficult part. Now write down three things that you have learnt that you are able to take back to your practice.

Conclusion

Whilst chronic pain management does require a range of resources to be most effective, you will have seen through your studies that there are a huge range of creative strategies that can be utilised in almost any caring environment. It does, however, require a regular commitment and a holistic approach that is patient- rather than disease-centred, and moves beyond the biomedical model that dominates care today. This is the real challenge for all staff and it is appropriate in the conclusion to focus on just why this is so important.

The biomedical model has the following features:

- It assumes that pain and other physical symptoms are the predominant cause of suffering in the dying.
- It carries a belief that these symptoms are best managed by establishing their root cause and by utilising modern pharmacology and other biomedical innovations for their 'relief'.
- The psychological, spiritual and social aspects of these symptoms, though considered important to be addressed, are of secondary rather than primary importance.

- Using the biomedical model to manage these problems has a tendency to objectify the problem and risks the denial of personhood and the decontextualisation of the problem.
- It can also risk the denial of chronic illness, suffering and meaning as part of the experience of illness and dying.

References

Becker, R. (2000) Competency assessment in palliative nursing. *European Journal of Palliative Care*, **7**(3), 88–91.

Benner, P. (1984) *From Novice to Expert: Excellence and Power in Clinical Practice*. Addison-Wesley, California.

Berkovitch, M., Waller, A. and Adunsky, A. (1999) High dose morphine use in the hospice setting: a database survey of patient characteristics and effect on life expectancy. *Cancer*, **86**(5), 871–7.

European Association for Palliative Care (1996). Morphine in cancer pain: modes of administration. Expert Working Group of the European Association for Palliative Care. *British Medical Journal*, **312**, 823–6.

Hanks, G. W., Conno, F. and Cherny, N. (2001) Expert Working Group of the Research Network of the European Association for Palliative Care: Morphine and Alternative opioids in cancer pain: the EAPC recommendations. *British Journal of Cancer*, **84**(5), 587–93.

Pargeon, K. L. and Hailey, B. J. (1999) Barriers to effective cancer pain management: a review of the literature. *Journal of Pain and Symptom Management*, **18**(5), 358–68.

Porta-Sales, J. *et al.* (2003). *European Journal of Palliative Care*, **10**(3), 105–9.

McCaffery, M. (1972) *Nursing Management of the Patient in Pain*. J. B. Lippincott, Philadelphia.

Regnard, C. F. B. and Tempest, S. (1998) *A Guide to Symptom Relief in Advanced Cancer*, 4th edn. Haigh and Hochland, Manchester.

Stevens, R. A. and Ghazi, S. M. (2000) Routes of opiod analgesic therapy in the management of cancer pain. *Cancer Control*, **7**(2), 131–41.

Royal College of Nursing (2002) *A Framework for Nurses Working in Specialist Palliative Care: Competencies Project*. RCN Publications, London.

World Health Organization (1986) *Cancer Pain Relief*. WHO, Geneva.

World Health Organization (1990) Cancer pain relief and palliative care. *Technical Report Series 804*. WHO, Geneva.

World Health Organization (1996) *Cancer Pain Relief with a Guide to Opioid Availability*. WHO, Geneva.

Original material for this chapter was taken and adapted from the Management of Pain online study course authored by R. Becker and available at: http://www.cancernursing.org/.

🖥 Useful websites

Scottish Intercollegiate Guidelines Network – pain control
http://www.sign.ac.uk/guidelines/fulltext/44/

Pain.com
http://www.pain.com/sections/categories_of_pain/cancer/

Cancer pain.org
http://www.cancer-pain.org/

Cancer pain management in children
http://www.childcancerpain.org/

Hospice Net
http://www.hospicenet.org/html/what_is_pain.html

The Oxford Pain internet Site
http://www.jr2.ox.ac.uk/bandolier/booth/painpag/

📋 Chapter links to the Nursing and Midwifery Council Standards of Conduct, Performance and Ethics for Nurses and Midwives (2008)

Section 1: Make the care of people your first concern, treating them as individuals and respecting their dignity

Treat people as individuals
- You must treat people as individuals and respect their dignity
- You must treat people kindly and considerately
- You must act as an advocate for those in your care, helping them to access relevant health and social care, information and support

Collaborate with those in your care
- You must listen to the people in your care and respond to their concerns and preferences
- You must support people in caring for themselves to improve and maintain their health
- You must recognise and respect the contribution that people make to their own care and wellbeing
- You must make arrangements to meet people's language and communication needs

- You must share with people, in a way they can understand, the information they want or need to know about their health

Ensure you gain consent
- You must ensure that you gain consent before you begin any treatment or care
- You must respect and support people's rights to accept or decline treatment and care
- You must uphold people's rights to be fully involved in decisions about their care
- You must be aware of the legislation regarding mental capacity, ensuring that people who lack capacity remain at the centre of decision making and are fully safeguarded

Section 2: Work with others to protect and promote the health and wellbeing of those in your care, their families and carers, and the wider community

Share information with your colleagues
- You must keep your colleagues informed when you are sharing the care of others

Work effectively as part of a team
- You must work cooperatively within teams and respect the skills, expertise and contributions of your colleagues
- You must consult and take advice from colleagues when appropriate
- You must make a referral to another practitioner when it is in the best interests of someone in your care

Section 3: Provide a high standard of practice and care at all times

Use the best available evidence
- You must deliver care based on the best available evidence or best practice.
- You must ensure any advice you give is evidence based if you are suggesting healthcare products or services
- You must ensure that the use of complementary or alternative therapies is safe and in the best interests of those in your care

Keep your skills and knowledge up to date
- You must have the knowledge and skills for safe and effective practice when working without direct supervision
- You must recognise and work within the limits of your competence

■ You must take part in appropriate learning and practice activities that maintain and develop your competence and performance

Keep clear and accurate records

■ You must keep clear and accurate records of the discussions you have, the assessments you make, the treatment and medicines you give and how effective these have been
■ You must complete records as soon as possible after an event has occurred
■ You must not tamper with original records in any way
■ You must ensure any entries you make in someone's paper records are clearly and legibly signed, dated and timed
■ You must ensure any entries you make in someone's electronic records are clearly attributable to you
■ You must ensure all records are kept confidentially and securely

☑ Self-assessment test

1. According to the WHO analgesic ladder, when should you move up to the next step of the analgesic ladder?
   A When pain is under control
   B No need to move up unless the pain experienced is severe
   C Move up if the pain is not controlled by proper doses of the drug at regular intervals
   D Move up if the drug has *not* been given at regular intervals

2. Which ONE of the following drugs is appropriate treatment for Step One of the analgesic ladder?
   A Tramadol
   B Codeine
   C Paracetamol
   D Diamorphine

3. Which combination drug is appropriate for Step Two of the WHO analgesic ladder?
   A Co-dydramol
   B Diamorphine
   C Aspirin
   D Methadone

4. Which ONE of the following drugs is *not* an opioid?
   A Methadone
   B Dextropopoxyphene
   C Diclofenac
   D Fentanyl

5. Which ONE of the following is *not* a principle of prescribing analgesics?
   A Prescribe analgesics according to the WHO ladder
   B Always prescribe an opioid in the first instance
   C Prescribe analgesics by mouth in the first instance
   D Analgesics should be administered regularly and sufficiently

6. Which ONE of the following statements is *not* one of the Ten Commandments of Good Pain Control?
   A Do take the patient's feelings into consideration at all times
   B Do assume the patient's pain is caused by the malignant process
   C Do prescribe adequate amounts of analgesia
   D Do not limit your approach to simply analgesics

7. Which ONE of the following statements is true?
   A Opioids alone can relieve all pain
   B Control of physical pain is the main priority
   C Elevating a patient's mood has no effect on physical pain
   D Analgesic drugs alone will not relieve all pain

8. Which ONE of the following side-effects is *rarely* seen in patients using opioids for chronic pain?
   A Constipation
   B Nausea
   C Respiratory depression
   D Vomiting

9. Which ONE of the following is the primary route of choice for administration of analgesics?
   A Sublingual
   B Oral
   C Transdermal
   D Subcutaneous

10. When a patient is unable to take oral medication due to nausea and vomiting, which *non-invasive* route of administration provides the quickest pain relief?
    A Epidural
    B Sublingual
    C Intravenous
    D Rectal

11. Which ONE of the following side-effects may require the dose of drug to be altered?
    A Dry mouth
    B Constipation
    C Sedation
    D Nausea

12. When is it appropriate to convert to controlled/sustained release drug preparations?
    A When the patient has severe or breakthrough pain
    B When ascertaining the patient's level of pain
    C During drug titration
    D When good pain relief has been achieved

13. Which ONE of the following is the best way to treat breakthrough pain?
    A Treat with an immediate supplementary dose of opioids
    B Treat with controlled release morphine
    C Wait 24 hours then increase the opioid dose
    D Treat with a dose of opioids the equivalent of the patient's normal daily prescription

14. Which ONE of the following is *not* part of good nursing practice?
    A Giving analgesia at an appropriate interval before a painful procedure
    B Administering breakthrough analgesia without explanation to the patient
    C Waiting 30 minutes to assess response of pain after breakthrough analgesia
    D Re-assessing total pain management if pain continuously persists

15.   What is the meaning of adjuvant drugs with regard to pain management?
    A Adjuvant drugs are used alone to treat severe pain
    B Adjuvant drugs can be used in place of opioids
    C Adjuvant drugs are used to treat pain before administering an opioid
    D Adjuvant drugs are used to aid the effectiveness of opioids

CHAPTER II

Managing symptoms other than pain

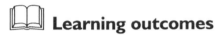 *I felt sick, I got a tablet, I couldn't breathe, I got another tablet. Now I can't go to the toilet. I watched the doctor write out another prescription. I hoped it would help but I was running out of faith. Along came Dawn. She asked me about everything and everything is now getting better.*

Learning outcomes

After reading this chapter and completing the reflective activities the learner will be able to:

- Identify the main symptoms that affect quality of life for the terminally ill
- Describe a range of approaches that are effective in symptom management
- Outline the nursing priorities when managing multiple symptomatology

Introduction

The short anecdote above tells us a lot about the place in which care is being delivered and also the staff within that area. It would be easy to criticise our medical colleague for not bothering to look at the effect that their prescriptions were having on the patient and for not noticing the concern the patient is expressing. Context is everything of course, and there are many busy acute care settings where such events are commonplace and it does not necessarily mean that people fail to care. It is more about the culture and pressures of the job at that moment. The more interesting part of this story is what happens next. Dawn is the nurse who put the humanity back into the care process: by using her listening and attending skills, her competence at putting the patient at ease and her skilled questioning technique she was able to ease the patient's distress. It was quite clear to Dawn that the nausea, the dyspnoea and the constipation were ongoing issues that merited attention and the doctor's prescription would hopefully help, but in that moment it was more important to attend to the needs of the whole person.

This chapter will examine the frequency of the most common symptoms experienced in advanced illness and outline their overall management. Although it is recognised that the medical interventions prescribed and thence delivered by nurses may well determine the overall outcome of care, the focus will be on the holistic nursing priorities, which can make a significant difference to quality of life – as the story of Dawn and her patient has shown.

Roper *et al.* (1980) said that the goal of nursing is to help patients to solve, alleviate or cope with problems they encounter. With all aspects of palliative care and notably symptom management other than pain we *may* be able to solve problems, but we also have to live with the fact that we *may* not. Recent pharmacological and non-pharmacological developments have given us many opportunities to extensively alleviate problems, but some remain intractable and difficult to improve, which is why we must never omit to help patients cope with their problems.

Nursing principles of symptom management

- Involve all appropriate members of the multidisciplinary team
- Meticulous holistic assessment: consider physical, psychological, spiritual and social factors
- Identify the patient's direct concerns before beginning the biochemical interventions
- Ask 'What can I do to help?' and 'What can my colleagues do to help?'
- Listen attentively without judgement
- Demonstrate empathy
- Explain the possible causes and the available treatment options
- Decide with the medical staff on the most appropriate treatment, considering both medical and non-medical interventions
- Set realistic goals with the patient and work hard at maintaining hope
- Be always vigilant for new symptoms and new causes for existing symptoms
- Review the situation regularly – at least every 24 hours

Frequency of common symptoms

The list below illustrates the frequency of common symptoms in advanced illness based on current evidence (Buckley, 2008).

- Pain
- Nausea and vomiting
- Constipation
- Diarrhoea
- Anorexia
- Fatigue
- Breathlessness
- Confusion
- Insomnia
- Anxiety
- Depression

Symptoms like these are all too often managed in isolation rather than understanding that patients frequently have multiple symptoms with multiple causes.

Reflective activity

Case study: Bill

Bill was a 70-year-old man with cancer of the prostate. After a couple of days in hospital his pain was well controlled with a combination of morphine and diclofenac. Bill complained of nausea when talking to one nurse. He was subsequently given metoclopramide, an anti-emetic. Later that day he told another nurse he had abdominal pain. A different doctor prescribed Maalox, an antacid. He was discharged home a few days later and visited by his community nursing auxiliary. Bill told her he was having some problem going to the toilet. The nurse told the doctor, who prescribed an antibiotic for a urinary tract infection.

The next day Sally, the community staff-nurse, went to see Bill. He appeared very unwell and perhaps depressed. Sally spent 15 minutes with him assessing his pain and all his symptoms. She reported back to the GP and suggested a joint visit.

What are the principal issues for Bill that need to be addressed? Make yourself a list and compare it to the feedback below.

Feedback

The joint visit took place the next day and the conclusions they reached were:

- Bill's nausea was due to the morphine he began taking a few days ago. He was given haloperidol for this with excellent effect.
- The abdominal pain was due to the diclofenac. His GP prescribed lansoprazole, which eased his pain two days later. Sally discussed Bill's eating habits and explained the importance of talking diclofenac with meals.
- When Sally asked him about, 'going to the toilet', Bill was a little embarrassed. He said, 'It's not my waterworks, it's the other'. Sally asked him how often he

was going to the toilet and if it was difficult. Bill said,' It's the piles, you know, they are very painful and it's very hard to go'. The GP examined Bill's anus and rectum. He found multiple haemorrhoids and a rectum full of hard faeces. Sally planned to come back later to give Bill a softening enema. The GP prescribed a stool softener and stimulant to treat the constipation. He also prescribed some ointment to reduce the pain and swelling around Bill's haemorrhoids. The antibiotic for Bill's non-existent urinary tract infection was stopped immediately.

Lessons to be learned
■ Patients commonly experience multiple symptoms. Assessing one symptom at a time may result in an incomplete assessment
■ Medications to treat one symptom frequently cause another. For example, opioids used to treat pain can cause constipation and nausea
■ Embarrassment on the part of the patient or professional may result in symptoms being overlooked
■ Listen to the patient
■ Review regularly

Sally continued to visit daily. Each day Bill's condition improved. On day five a smiling Bill greeted her at the door. He had no pain, nausea or constipation. Sally agreed to visit every few days to monitor these symptoms and to look for the development of anything new.

The remainder of the chapter will discuss the management of the most common symptoms encountered.

Assessment tools

There are a wide range of published assessment tools available to measure symptom distress and quality of life, and it is appropriate to mention a few of the best.

■ **The Support Team Assessment Schedule (STAS)** (Higginson, 1993). This tool was originally designed in the UK for use in community settings and has a 17 item inventory of questions covering a range of areas from pain and symptoms, psychosocial issues, family needs, insight into the illness, communication, home services and the support of other professionals. It is still widely used as it is quick (2–3 minutes; so does not tire the patient) and comprehensive.

- **The Rotterdam Symptom Checklist (RSCL)** (De Haes *et al.*, 1990). This 34 item inventory can be used to assess a range of both physical and psychosocial problems. Because of its length it is not so widely used today.
- **The Palliative Care Outcome Scale (PCOS)** (Hearn and Higginson, 1999). This tool is a straightforward 10 point questionnaire for use by both staff and patients.
- **The Palliative Care Assessment Tool (PCAT)** (Ellershaw *et al.*, 1995). This has a quick numerical scoring system that can used with the patient and covers a wide range of symptomatology. According to Conner and Muir (2007) it has proved very reliable in clinical practice and can be used with any symptom.

The pick of the choices here for nurses caring for patients in busy environments is the last one on the list (PCAT; Table 11.1). It has been extensively evaluated in practice, is seen to be very reliable and the simple scoring system, which can be universally applied to any symptom, makes it a practical and useful tool.

Table 11.1 The Palliative Care Assessment Tool.

Problem absent = 0
Problem present, but not affecting the patient's day = 1
Problem present and having a moderate effect on the patient's day = 2
Problem present and dominating the patients day = 3

Nausea and vomiting

Nausea is a very unpleasant feeling, familiar to us all, whereas vomiting is the act of being sick. Patients with advanced illness say that nausea is much worse than vomiting.

Vomiting mechanism

Vomiting is controlled by the vomiting centre in the brain. It is activated by stimuli from:

- The chemoreceptor trigger zone (CTZ)
- The upper gastrointestinal tract and pharynx

- The vestibular apparatus
- Higher centres in the cerebral cortex triggered by sounds, smells worries and associations, for example when the chemotherapy appointment arrives

Causes of vomiting

There is a single cause in two-thirds of patients.

- CTZ
  - Drugs such as opioids, chemotherapy, tricyclic antidepressants
  - Biochemical reasons such as hypercalcaemia, raised urea, and renal and hepatic failure
- Vestibular
  - Tumour
  - Opioids
  - Inner ear disturbance
- Cerebral cortex
  - Anxiety
  - Raised intracranial pressure
  - Association and previous experience
- Peripheral
  - Radiotherapy
  - Chemotherapy
  - Gastrointestinal irritation by pressure, inflammation or obstruction

Principles of management

Selecting appropriate anti-emetic drugs is essential. So are the other measures listed below:

- Ensure patient privacy
- Identify and treat the cause if possible
- Manage the environment: reduce unpleasant smells; careful, sensitive explanation
- Offer mouthwashes and preferred fluids in small amounts
- Facilities to wash hands and face
- Empty and replace vomit bowl immediately after vomiting. A large bowl is much better than a small 'kidney dish'
- Measuring fluid balance may be necessary in protracted vomiting

■ Optimise non-pharmacological measures
■ Review at least every 24 hours

Always ask yourself 'What is the likely cause of nausea and vomiting in this particular patient?'

Anti-emetic therapy

■ Anticipate the need and give well before emetogenic stimulus
■ Use adequate and regular doses
■ Use appropriate route(s)
■ Aim at the appropriate receptor(s)
■ Combine drugs if more than one cause exists but keep regime as simple as possible

Features and management of nausea and vomiting by cause

1. Gastric stasis
Features: Patient feels full. Often only slightly nauseated before vomiting. Vomit may be large and patient feels better after vomiting.

Management: If possible discontinue contributory medication or reduce dose. A prokinetic drug will help, for example metoclopramide.

2. Intestinal obstruction
Features: Uncomfortable abdominal distension, generally unwell, may have colic. Large volume vomit is common. NB: it may be possible to treat the obstruction surgically. A surgical opinion should be sought.

Management: If no colic is present, subcutaneous metoclopramide and a faecal softener. If colic is present, subcutaneous cyclizine and hyoscine butyl-bromide together with a faecal softener.

3. Biochemical disturbance
Features: Gradual onset with constant symptoms, such as fatigue, confusion, weakness, anorexia and constipation. Nausea is usually constant.

Management: If possible and appropriate, correct the biochemical distur-bance with subcutaneous haloperidol.

4. Drugs
Features: There may be little to find on examination. Careful observation will reveal the relationship between consumption of drug and nausea.

- Anticholinergics, chlorpromazine and opioids can cause **gastric stasis** Treat with **metoclopramide**.
- NSAIDs, ampicillin, erythromycin, iron supplements and some cytotoxics can cause **gastric irritation**. Treat with **metoclopramide**.
- Opioids, anticonvulsants, trimethoprim, metronidazole, ketoconazole, cytotoxics and some anaesthetic agents affect the **CTZ**. Treat with**haloperidol**.
- **NB**: some drugs not noted for causing nausea may cause nausea in some patients. Listen to the patient and believe them.

5. Raised ICP

Features: Onset may be gradual or sudden. Sensation of nausea may fluctuate. Neurological features such as paralysis, aphasia, amnesia and depression.

Management: Steroids help by reducing oedema around the tumour. Cyclizine. Consider the possibility of radiotherapy, surgery or a shunt.

Constipation

> When I got up this morning I took two Ex-Lax in addition to my Prozac.
> I can't get off the toilet, but at least I feel good about it.

Constipation is a very common problem in advanced disease, especially in patients taking opioids or with neurological disease. It can mimic the signs of advanced disease. It is embarrassing for patients to discuss; therefore tact and diplomacy are required. In advanced disease it does not usually respond to exercise, increased fluid and fibre intake. Laxatives are almost always required.

What is constipation?

Constipation must never be defined by frequency of bowel action alone. It has been described as infrequent or difficult defaecation caused by decreased intestinal motility or a decrease in the frequency of the passage of formed stool characterised by stools that are hard and difficult to pass.

Signs and symptoms of constipation

- Difficulty in passing stool
- Generalised or colicky abdominal pain

- Distended abdomen
- Flatulence
- Anorexia and nausea
- Increased or absent bowel sounds
- Confusion
- Diarrhoea: this should always be investigated. It may be due to loose stools bypassing hard faeces in the rectum. Treating with agents which firm the stool will make matters considerably worse. A digital rectal examination is essential.

Common causes of constipation

- Direct effects of cancer
- Obstruction
- Neurological damage
- Hypercalcaemia
- Secondary effects of advanced illness
- Poor dietary and fluid intake
- Weakness and immobility
- Poor/unfamiliar toilet arrangements
- Confusion
- Drugs: opioids, tricyclic antidepressants, anti-Parkinsonian agents, phenothiazines, hyoscine, diuretics, anticonvulsants, iron anti-hypertensives
- Hypothyroidism
- Hypokalaemia
- Diabetes
- Diverticular disease
- Haemorrhoids, anal fissures/stenosis
- Rectocele
- Colitis

Assessment

- Sensitivity and *privacy*
- Discuss associated symptoms
- Identify normal bowel patterns: frequency; 'What is it like when you "go to the toilet"?'
- Usual bowel habits and changes in habits
- Drug regimes (prescribed and over the counter)

- Worries and concerns: constipation can mimic advanced abdominal cancer
- Toilet facilities and 'after toilet' facilities: disposal and hand-washing
- Digital rectal examination
- Abdominal X-ray
- *Remember*: frequency of bowel action alone is *not* a reliable indicator of constipation

Management of constipation

- Prevention of constipation is easier than treatment and should be the management strategy
- Regular bowel chart. This may appear 'old fashioned', but it can provide useful information
- Attention to diet. Maximise fluid and fibre intake
- Increase mobility
- Treatment of correctable causes
- Laxatives
- Home planning: modification may help
- Mouth care
- Food, fluids and supplements
- Education: explain about need to take medication regularly

Manual evacuation

This procedure is occasionally necessary. Some paraplegic patients develop a regime whereby their stools are kept reasonably firm and they require manual evacuation every 2 or 3 days, but it is an unpleasant and undignified procedure. Skilled nursing will minimise distress. Careful explanation is essential. Some hospices carry out this procedure with sedation in very ill patients. The patient is given intravenous midazolam, which has a sedative and amnesic action

Laxatives

Should be given prophylactically. They usually have a softening, lubricant, stimulant or combined action. As with opioids, dose titration is important. Some patients prefer laxatives they have become accustomed to and this can aid compliance. Patients and carers need education so that they understand the principles of preventing constipation.

Most laxatives are well tolerated. Patients may be alarmed if they have red urine after taking Danthron. It may also cause peri-anal skin irritation. Lactulose is safe and popular. Its sweet taste can be unpleasant for some and it may cause a feeling of fullness or cause colic. If constipation is caused by opioids, lactulose and senna appear to be equally effective but senna may be too 'severe' for some, causing griping abdominal pain.

Rectal preparations

Suppositories and enemas are sometimes required if other methods are ineffective. They should be avoided if at all possible. Careful explanation is needed so that patients know when to retain rectal preparations. The patients must be within easy access of toilet facilities. If they are weak help must be available.

Breathlessness

This can be a terrifying symptom, with patients fearing death is near. Approximately one third of cancer patients and 70% of lung cancer patients will experience breathlessness. It is common in patients with chronic obstructive pulmonary disease (COPD) and cardiac failure. Patients may experience a sensation of suffocation, poor concentration, loss of appetite, loss of memory, profuse sweating and a feeling of isolation.

Common causes

- Primary tumour occluding an airway
- Metastatic spread
- Lymphatic occlusion
- COPD
- Asthma
- Pleural effusion
- Pulmonary embolus
- Anaemia
- Pneumothorax
- Chest infection

■ Cardiac failure
■ Renal failure leading to generalised oedema
■ Fear and anxiety
■ Superior vena cava obstruction

Management

Begin with a detailed assessment of breathlessness and factors which ameliorate or exacerbate it. Discuss and explain the meaning of breathlessness and its place in the illness. Patients often regard breathlessness as an inevitable consequence of lung cancer. Provide advice and support on methods of managing breathlessness for the patients and their family. A specialist nurse or physiotherapist can teach breathing retraining, relaxation and distraction, while all nurses can help with goal setting to learn helpful techniques and integrate them into daily life. Early recognition of problems that may need drug treatment is important and general advice on maintaining health will optimise care.

First consider simple but effective measures. Change the patient's position. They may prefer to sit upright in a bed or chair supported by pillows. Circulating air reduces the subjective feeling of breathlessness. Open a window and provide a fan. Reduce overcrowding from staff and visitors to provide a calm atmosphere. Touch may relieve anxiety and relaxation exercises may help further. Plan the patient's day to conserve energy. Simple breathing exercises will help. Encourage the patient to breathe *out* slowly. It is frightening to be told to breathe slowly if you are fighting for breath. Involve the entire team where appropriate. A home assessment will reveal where additional equipment, nursing and social care will help. A specialist nurse, doctor or psychologist may help if anxiety and panic attacks are troublesome. Cognitive behavioural therapy can help in severe panic attacks.

Medication

■ Benzodiazepines such as diazepam, lorazepam and midazolam can bring symptomatic relief
■ Small doses of oral morphine can help reduce the sensation of breathlessness. Morphine acts centrally to diminish the ventilatory drive stimulated by hypercapnia, hypoxia, and exercise
■ Nebulised opioids act through a central as opposed to a local pulmonary mechanism. This is a relatively inefficient way of administering morphine
■ Steroids may reduce swelling around the tumour.

Oxygen has been shown to improve exercise tolerance and prolong life in patients with COPD who are severely hypoxic. This may be due to the placebo effect, but the cooling flow of oxygen against the face or through the nose may reduce breathlessness. Some patients keep an oxygen supply at the top and bottom of their stairs at home. Unfortunately, patients may become psychologically dependent on oxygen, to such an extent that they are unable to go anywhere without it (Bredin *et al.*, 1999).

Weakness and fatigue

Weakness and fatigue are common debilitating symptoms in advanced illness. The presence of other symptoms, such as pain and nausea, exacerbates weakness and fatigue and adversely affect patients' quality of life.

Possible causes of generalised weakness and fatigue

- Anaemia
- Drugs
- Sepsis
- Metabolic imbalance
- Cardiac, respiratory and renal failure
- Lack of sleep and rest
- Exhaustion due to the sheer weight of coping with the illness
- Poor nutritional intake
- Dehydration
- Depression
- Stress
- Overactivity

Possible causes of localised weakness

- Localised trauma
- Nerve damage
- Spinal cord compression
- Brain metastases
- Neuropathy due to drug therapy

Management of weakness and fatigue

- Meticulous assessment
- Team approach particularly physiotherapist and occupational therapist
- Treat reversible causes such as anaemia and electrolyte imbalance
- Enhance food and fluid intake
- Review medications
- Gentle exercise can enhance wellbeing
- Careful planning of the patient's environment and day
- Plan rest periods throughout day and enhance sleep
- Use aids to reduce energy expenditure. A wheelchair allows patients to 'scull' around home/ward and reduce energy expenditure
- Set realistic goals
- Steroids may provide short- or long-term benefit

Anxiety and depression

There is a common misconception that anxiety and depression are inevitable consequences of advanced illness. Anxiety and depression do not always occur together, but they are discussed together here.

Common causes of anxiety and depression

- Pre-existing mental health problems
- Marital or relationship problems, such as divorce and separation
- Financial worries
- Fear of illness, pain, loss, needles, chemotherapy or death itself
- Lack of support from family and professionals
- Drugs with an adrenaline-like action, such as salbutamol

Questions to ask

- Can you tell me how you are feeling?
- Do you know why you feel this way?
- Do you have specific worries or concerns?
- What do you think is going to happen to you?

- How are you sleeping?
- What do you think has caused you to feel this way?
- Do you always feel so low or does it come and go?
- How long have you felt like this?
- Do you find you have lost interest in things around you?
- Do you have any feelings of guilt? If so, can you tell me about them?
- What brought these feelings on?

If a patient says or hints they are feeling suicidal it must be taken seriously. They may have a treatable depression. They may actually have considered taking their own life. Clearly you must pass on your findings to a colleague, but remain supportive of the patient. You may ask:

- Have you actually thought about taking your own life? If the answer is yes you may carefully explore how the patient has considered taking their life. This will not encourage them to commit suicide.
- Does anyone else know you feel this way?
- What might we do to help you feel better?

Drug treatment

Anxiety may be managed using small doses of benzodiazepines such as diazepam, midazolam or lorazepam. Beta blockers such as propanolol can reduce the subjective feeling of anxiety by blocking the action of adrenaline.

Depression is commonly treated with selective serotonin-reuptake inhibitors such as fluoexetine (Prozac). Older antidepressant drugs, for example tricyclic antidepressants such as amitriptyline, can be of benefit. All antidepressant have side effects. The gains must always be weighed against the possible benefits. Perceived prognosis is sometimes used as a reason for not prescribing antidepressant medications because they are not effective immediately. Judging prognosis is notoriously difficult; therefore they should not be withheld without meticulous assessment and planning involving the patient.

Non-drug measures

- Drugs offer symptomatic relief in the management of anxiety and depression. Some causes can be addressed and relieved. The continued presence of staff who will stay with the patient through difficult times offers continued hope.

- Acknowledge the anxiety and provide someone to talk to, someone who will listen, someone who will give time.
- Discuss the reasons for anxiety and depression
- Simple jargon-free advice. It can be enormously helpful to know that a new pain is a muscle strain and not cancer which has spread.
- Distraction: something to do
- Rest and sleep
- The support and advice of a community psychiatric nurse, GP, psychologist or psychiatrist
- Counselling
- Psychotherapy
- Cognitive behavioural therapy

Conclusion

The management of symptoms other than pain is a complex business, and the prescription of appropriate medication, whilst a medical role, is very much complemented by the vitally important role of the nurse. It is nurses who have the most contact with the patient and are in the best position to notice changes in their condition and to be both proactive in the planning of care to avoid the worst of such symptomatology and quickly reactive to presenting symptoms to help minimise distress. Careful and regular assessment combined with a holistic approach is the key to success.

References

Buckley, J. (2008) Eleven prevalent symptoms. In *Palliative Care: an Integrated Approach*. Wiley, Blackwell, Chichester.

Bredin, M., Corner, J., Krishnasamy, M., Plant, H., Bailey, C. and A'Hern, R. (1999) Multicentre randomised controlled trial of nursing intervention for breathlessness in patients with lung cancer. *British Medical Journal*, **318**, 901–4.

Conner, A. and Muire, M. (2007) Managing symptoms: what can nurses do? A principle based approach. In: Palliative Nursing; Improving End of Life Care, 2nd edn (eds. S. Kinghorn and S. Gaines). Churchill Livingstone Elsevier, London.

De Haes, J. C., Van Knippenberg, F. C. and Neijt, J. P. (1990) measuring psychological and physical distress in cancer patients: structure and application of the Rotterdam Symptom checklist. *British Journal of Cancer*, **62**, 1034–8.

Ellershaw, J. E., Peat, S. J. and Boys, L. C. (1995) Assessing the effectiveness of a hospital palliative care team. *Palliative Medicine*, **9**(2), 145–52.

Hearn, J. and Higginson, I. (1999) Development and validation of a care outcome masure for palliative care: the Palliative Care Outcome Scale, Palliative Care Audit Project Advisory Group. *Quality in Health Care*, **8**(4), 219–27.

Higginson, I. (1993) A community schedule. In: *Clinical Audit in Palliative Care* (ed. I. Higginson). Radcliffe Medical Press, Oxford.

Hill, S. (2000) Symptom control. In: Stepping into Palliative Care. A Handbook for Community Professionals (ed. J. Cooper). Radcliffe Medical Press, Oxford.

Roper, N., Logan, W. and Tierney, A. (1980) *The Elements of Nursing*. Churchill Livingstone, Edinburgh.

 Useful websites

Managing Constipation in Advanced Illness
http://www.albertapalliative.net/APN/PCHB/06_Constipation.html
http://www.painconsult.com/Pcc4.htm

Dyspnoea
http://www.in-touch.org.uk/Dyspnoea%20Case%20History%20Master.htm
http://www.vtsm.co.uk/data/clinical/decisions/guidelines_palliative_care.htm#Dyspnoea

Nausea and vomiting
http://www.jr2.ox.ac.uk/bandolier/booth/booths/pall.html
http://bmj.com/cgi/content/full/315/7116/1148
http://www.sea-band.com/The%20Sea%20Band/health.htm

Lymphoedema
http://www.lymphoedema.org/
http://www.cclf.co.uk/
http://www.cancerbacup.org.uk/info/lymphedema.htm

Depression
http://www.psychiatry.ox.ac.uk/cebmh/elmh/depression/index.html
http://www.psychiatry.ox.ac.uk/cebmh/elmh/depression/bibliography/index.html
http://cebmh.warne.ox.ac.uk/cebmh/whoguidemhpcuk/leaflets/07-1.html

Bowel obstruction
http://hospice.xtn.net//obstruct/

✍ Chapter links to the Nursing and Midwifery Council Standards of Conduct, Performance and Ethics for Nurses and Midwives (2008)

Section 1: Make the care of people your first concern, treating them as individuals and respecting their dignity

Treat people as individuals
- You must treat people as individuals and respect their dignity
- You must treat people kindly and considerately
- You must act as an advocate for those in your care, helping them to access relevant health and social care, information and support

Respect people's confidentiality
- You must respect people's right to confidentiality
- You must ensure people are informed about how and why information is shared by those who will be providing their care
- You must disclose information if you believe someone may be at risk of harm, in line with the law of the country in which you are practising

Collaborate with those in your care
- You must listen to the people in your care and respond to their concerns and preferences
- You must support people in caring for themselves to improve and maintain their health
- You must recognise and respect the contribution that people make to their own care and wellbeing
- You must make arrangements to meet people's language and communication needs
- You must share with people, in a way they can understand, the information they want or need to know about their health

Ensure you gain consent
- You must ensure that you gain consent before you begin any treatment or care
- You must respect and support people's rights to accept or decline treatment and care
- You must uphold people's rights to be fully involved in decisions about their care
- You must be aware of the legislation regarding mental capacity, ensuring that people who lack capacity remain at the centre of decision making and are fully safeguarded

Section 2: Work with others to protect and promote the health and wellbeing of those in your care, their families and carers, and the wider community

Share information with your colleagues
- You must keep your colleagues informed when you are sharing the care of others

Work effectively as part of a team
- You must consult and take advice from colleagues when appropriate
- You must make a referral to another practitioner when it is in the best interests of someone in your care

Section 3: Provide a high standard of practice and care at all times

Use the best available evidence
- You must deliver care based on the best available evidence or best practice.

Keep your skills and knowledge up to date
- You must have the knowledge and skills for safe and effective practice when working without direct supervision
- You must recognise and work within the limits of your competence
- You must take part in appropriate learning and practice activities that maintain and develop your competence and performance

Keep clear and accurate records
- You must keep clear and accurate records of the discussions you have, the assessments you make, the treatment and medicines you give and how effective these have been
- You must complete records as soon as possible after an event has occurred

☑ Self-assessment test

1. Which of these symptoms is the most common in advanced illness?
   A Vomiting and nausea
   B Breathlessness
   C Pain
   D Constipation

2. The Patient Care Assessment Tool (PCAT) is seen by many as the best assessment tool for symptom distress because:
    A It is the most academically rigorous
    B It is reliable, simple and easy to use
    C It is readily available
    D It covers the widest range of symptoms

3. When managing nausea and vomiting you should always:
    A Tell the patient 'it will pass'
    B Promote fluids
    C Review the situation at least every 24 hours
    D Open the nearest window to allow fresh air in to disperse bad smells

4. Constipation can best be managed by a combination of:
    A Diet, mobility, manual evacuation
    B Laxatives, fluids, fruit
    C Enema, education, bowel chart
    D Treatment of correctable causes, high fibre intake, laxatives

5. Nursing priorities of breathlessness include:
    A Good supportive positioning
    B Education about simple breathing exercises
    C The use of small doses of oral morphine and nebulised morphine
    D All of the above

CHAPTER 12

Spiritual care

 The old grey donkey Eeyore stood by himself in a thistly corner of the forest, his front feet well apart, his head on one side and thought about things. Sometimes he thought sadly to himself 'Why?' and sometimes he thought 'Where?' and sometimes he didn't quite know what he was thinking about (Milne, 1992)

Learning outcomes

After reading this chapter and completing the reflective activities the learner will be able to:

- Understand the nature and meaning of spiritual care from a palliative perspective
- Utilise a range of strategies to promote spiritual care in a range of environments
- Reflect on personal values and beliefs and how these can influence nursing practice

Introduction

If, like Eeyore, you have ever asked yourself the questions Why me? Why this? and Why now? in the midst of a life crisis (and for certain we all have) then it may surprise you to know that it could be argued that you were in some way being spiritual. Whether you have a formal belief that guides your life, or not, we all need to find meaning and perspective to major events in our lives and there is no greater life crisis than facing our mortality. It is this that makes spiritual care such an important and integral concept in all nursing practice, but it is particularly focused in a palliative care context.

We ask the question – why, not because we anticipate a voice coming out of the air and giving us an answer, but because we are trying to make some rational sense of a complex and highly emotive event. Mostly we ask these profound questions of ourselves, but occasionally nurses and other health professionals are the ones on the receiving end. Once again it's important to remember that the person voicing these questions knows perfectly well that there is no rational answer and they are not expecting one. They nevertheless still feel an overwhelming need to voice it. It is this unique facet of humanity to contemplate our own existence and ask questions about it that makes us who we are and is why the skills necessary to support everyone in such a crisis are so important.

Definitions

Nursing literature offers a wide variety of definitions of both spirituality and religion, and for the most part there is agreement that the relationship between spirituality and conventional religious belief is confused and ambiguous. It is hardly surprising therefore that most nurses find interpreting and delivering such a sensitive area of nursing care a major challenge. Indeed, McSherry and Draper (1997) argue that to address spirituality adequately, nurses need to be self-aware, mature and introspective. They comment that these elements are a major barrier, since individuals will need to explore areas of their lives that are sacred, private and deeply personal. Equally. Kristeller *et al.* (1999) argue that the majority of general nurses feel that spiritual issues are neglected because of time constraints, a lack of confidence in managing these issues and role uncertainty.

It has also been argued that fear may be a reason for nurses' reluctance to incorporate spiritual care into practice: fear of getting into a situation that they cannot handle, fear of intruding on a patient's privacy, and fear of being converted or confused in their own belief system (Granstrom, 1990).

It is certainly true that nurses generally find spiritual healthcare hard to articulate because it raises so many questions about life in which there are no specific answers or probable certainties, and part of the problem is perhaps rooted in the language used to describe spiritual care and needs. By its very nature it is inherently profound and philosophical, sometimes religious in orientation, and almost invariably ancient in its foundation. It is often therefore both unfamiliar and difficult language for many people to use in conversation, especially at times of stress.

Becker (2001) argues that we should perhaps be trying to develop a more appropriate and acceptable vocabulary that represents spirituality as a caring concept: a vocabulary that is representative of contemporary language with the use of metaphors and phrases that don't induce the 'cringe' factor and without the use of slang or colloquialisms. This would not only help patients and families, it would also help the professionals who work with the dying in whatever setting, as they themselves find it just as difficult to understand and approach spiritual matters in their jobs, due in part to the vocabulary (Ross, 1994).

Despite these acknowledged difficulties there is clear evidence to suggest that the meeting of spiritual needs can improve the physical wellbeing of patients (McSherry, 2007). Many patients also state that attention to the spiritual side of their life adds to their well being and can even counteract some of the more negative aspects of illness (Catterall *et al.*, 1998).

Reflective point

There is a common misconception that in order to meet spiritual needs a nurse needs either to have a religious belief themselves, or to have undergone some special training to deliver complicated interventions (Kemp, 1999). The reality according to Ross (1996) is that there is no evidence to suggest that nurses who had been taught spiritual care were any better at doing it. It appears that the personal characteristics of the nurse seemed to determine the spiritual care they gave.

We can we learn from this that delivering spiritual care is clearly integral to who we are, our values, beliefs, personality and interpersonal skills. Seen in this context it has a place in clinical practice for all nurses in what ever setting. We know, however, that it is particularly focused on the dying, who regardless of culture, belief or background are common in their search for a meaningful context to the crushing emotional and physical dilemmas posed by terminal illness.

No formal definition of spiritual care will be offered in this book for the reasons stated at the beginning of this chapter. However, it is appropriate to share with you one of the simplest and most understandable statements ever uttered in this context to help you to gain a clear sense of the reality of spiritual care. These words come direct from the mouth of Canon Ian Ainsworth Smith, who is a chaplain at a major London teaching hospital, and are reproduced with permission. When asked for his own interpretation of spirituality and spiritual care he said:

> Spiritual care... can help provide either a lot of answers to profound questions, or provide a context in which a person can safely ask lots of difficult questions. There are not necessarily any answers, but we can learn to stay with the questions. Spiritual care can be described as how someone puts together your past, your present, and any future life you may have and what this means to you.

Notice how this statement avoids the use of formal religious language and talks about the skills, knowledge and behaviours needed to address spiritual care. It is also totally person-centred and acknowledges the subjective and profound nature of such care.

Nurses are frequently polarised in their approaches to the spiritual dimension and tend to adopt one or other of the following stances:

- Spiritual care is defined as a purely psychosocial problem, where all so-called spiritual needs can be explained by reference to psychological and sociological theory.
- The existence of any concept which considers spirituality is denied totally and patient needs defined in this way are avoided.
- Acknowledge the relevance of caring for the spirit as an important part of care and worthy of independent theory and consideration.

Reflective activity

Which point of view do you subscribe to and why? Make some notes in your portfolio and consider whether your answer is truly honest and perhaps influenced by other considerations, such as the loss of someone close to you, or the beliefs of someone you know well.

Our patients are facing the reality of dealing with their mortality as an everyday experience and unless we have been there ourselves, it is very difficult to understand the thoughts, feelings and behaviours that are dominant at such a time. We all try to find some meaning in the midst of a major life crisis and the challenge of searching for that meaning can be hard, for example:

- A person who has placed their faith in modern science and medicine to provide all the answers will feel let down and disappointed when told 'We cannot cure you'.
- A person who has lived their whole life doing good for others and who has a strong faith believing that God will reward them in times of difficulty can have their faith seriously undermined by the experience of enduring a potentially terminal illness.
- A person whose philosophy tells them that the material world is all that there is, and when it's your turn to die, that's it, can be very surprised when they find himself saying 'Why me? What does it all mean?' and 'Is there something more?'.

Reflective point

There is an old army adage from the First World War which says that when you are deep in the trenches and about to go over the top and face the gunfire with your comrades there is no such thing as an atheist. What do you think the meaning is behind this? And is it relevant to the three people described in the bullet points above?

Reflective activity

Case study: Harry

Harry is 63 years old, married with three grown-up children. He is a fork lift truck driver in a local factory and has a strong Christian faith. He has a diagnosis of carcinoma of the lung and is being treated with radiotherapy in the oncology ward of his local hospital. A student goes to his bedside one morning and he angrily says to her 'Why me? Why has God let this happen to me?'. He is bitter towards life in general and also towards the members of his church community, where he has been a lay reader for some years, as no one has come to visit him.

How can you help address the spiritual needs of someone like Harry? The chances are that you are now saying to yourself 'I haven't a clue'.

Here is a suggested strategy.

Problem: Spiritual distress and anger due to questioning of his faith

Care plan: Build trust and a good rapport with Harry

                Listen carefully to his anxieties and encourage him to talk about his needs

                Adopt a non-judgemental and empathic approach

                Ask his permission to contact the clergy in charge of his church to arrange a visit or someone else he has confidence in

                Ask if he wishes to see the hospital chaplain

We meet people like Harry on a daily basis, but struggle to know what to put on a care plan. As you can see, this care plan is simple and achievable. I once saw written under the subheading of 'Spiritual care' the words 'likes a gin and tonic after her meals'. This was in a specialist palliative care unit which had a strong holistic focus to care, which demonstrates that even experienced and so called 'experts' sometimes find it hard to express in acceptable words the spiritual dimension.

Universality

Spiritual needs can be said to be universal to all humankind and if that is accepted then they can embody a vast range of qualities, values and activities. Below are just a few that have been cited, and include the need:

- to love and to be loved
- to achieve a sense of purpose and meaning in our life
- to keep a sense of identity, individual value and worth
- to maintain a sense of realistic hope in life
- to fulfil relationships with people who matter to us
- to express our personal sexuality in terms of appearance
- valuing the importance of truth, freedom and responsibility
- to engage in meaningful work
- to be creative in our life
- to enjoy abstract, aesthetic pleasures which give personal meaning

 Reflective activity

You may agree with some of these and disagree with others. Ask yourself, however, how many of these apply in your life at the moment? You may be somewhat surprised at how many do.

Formality

Religious needs are specific to those people who have a definitive faith that supports and guides their life and can include the need:

- for individual and corporate worship
- to engage in personal and corporate prayer
- to take part in birth, maturation, marriage and death rituals
- for meditation and private contemplation
- to see a religious person who represents their faith
- to visit holy places
- to possess holy items which assist in the expression of faith
- to follow a religious vocation if desired

 Reflective activity

If you have a personal faith many of these will apply to you. If you do not have a personal faith scan down the list and ask yourself if any are relevant to you in your life. As with the previous list and activity, you may be somewhat surprised at how many do.

Profound questions

Many patients express their spiritual needs by asking seemingly impossible questions. As stated in the introduction to this chapter, these questions are mostly rhetorical in nature, and do not necessarily demand an explanatory response. They include questions like:

- How will I die?
- Will I be alone?
- Will I suffer?
- Why me?
- Is my illness some sort of punishment?
- I can't understand how I am feeling
- Am I behaving as I should?
- Is there a god at all?
- I don't have a faith?
- Am I being a hypocrite looking for god's help?
- Will anyone take me seriously?
- Will people tell me the truth?

If you have ever encountered these questions and stayed with a patient trying to support them then you have delivered spiritual care. You may well have walked away feeling inadequate and unsure whether you have helped the person or not or indeed questioning your own stance in this area. It is suggested that in order to better judge our competence in this area it is important that we ask of ourselves some questions. Below are some suggested questions that are for most of us eminently answerable.

- What do I value in my life?
- How do I find/get meaning in my life and work?
- Have I ever considered this subject myself and where do I stand?

 Reflective activity

There are some words used today in the context of spirituality that consistently cause confusion. It's important therefore that we understand their meaning, because they are likely to be used by some patients in a discussion surrounding beliefs. Find a good dictionary and look up and make a note of the definitions of the following words:

Agnostic, atheist, secular, humanist, pagan

Here are some suggestions of questions to ask to assist in discovering a patient's spiritual needs. The list is not exhaustive; it is merely a guide and can be supplemented by your own questions.

- How have you coped with your illness up to now?
- What are your thoughts while facing this difficulty?
- What is the hardest part of this for you?
- What else is happening in your life now?
- Has being ill brought about any new insights into your life?
- What is your biggest fear?

Notice the use of **how** and **what** once more to frame an open question which will encourage a conversational response.

Some more general questions that are not so direct and centre in on a review of the person's life include:

- Tell me about your life.
- What has happened to you?
- What have you done in your life that you feel good about?
- What has been the happiest part of your life?
- What challenges and difficulties have you had to face?

Replying to the responses to these questions is equally difficult; therefore here are some reflective and empathic responses that may be appropriate

- This must be really hard for you.
- As I listen I can sense your distress.
- Whatever you are feeling is understandable given the situation you are facing.

 ## Reflective activity

Case study: Hugh

Hugh is a 40-year-old school teacher and is married with two young children. He has been admitted to hospital in the latter stages of prostate cancer. He is a quiet and reserved man who likes classical music and has no expressed faith. He is extremely worried about what will happen to his wife and children when he dies and is frustrated by his weakness and loss of independence and control over his life.

How can you help address the spiritual needs of someone like Harry? Below is a suggested plan.

Problem: Anxiety due to concerns over the future security of his family

Care plan: Encourage him to talk about his feelings

Help him to review his plans for his family and to set new goals

Problem: Feels helpless because of his illness and loss of independence
Care plan: Foster realistic hope by helping him focus on the achievements in his life and happy events that give meaning to him
Encourage him to use his family as a source of strength

Problem: Needs an opportunity for relaxation
Care plan: Explore the possibility of his family bringing in a music player so that he can listen to his favourite classical music

Hugh may not have an expressed faith, but as you can see there is a lot we can do to help him. Remember that a range of factors may influence how we both interpret and deliver spiritual care, namely the nurse, the carer, the culture and structure of the organisation, the characteristics of the patient and the family or loved ones. There are many routes to good spiritual care, some of which are simple and within the capacity of all nurses, whatever their education or background.

Nursing strategies

- Stay with the person; be with them and alongside them. Know when to stop *doing* and start *being*.
- Listen to them and hear the pain. Being heard and accepted in the depths of despair may lift spirits and is part of sharing with sensitivity and compassion.
- Drop your own agenda, because that gets in the way of unconditional care.
- Review your own beliefs, options and biases.
- Encourage them to express their fear and anger, i.e. give them permission.
- Provide a secure and caring environment which emphasises the patients needs as they see them.
- Reassure them about physical pain with information and practical help as desired and appropriate.
- Help them to spend time with those who matter to them.
- Help them to spend time alone and in a peaceful environment.
- Use appropriate fun and humour as patients greatly appreciate this aspect of normality.
- Review and remember with photos and mementos.
- Provide for religious and sacramental care with the appropriate minister for communion, prayer, confession or anointing if requested.

- Remember that the small, but important aesthetic things in life can make a huge difference, such as:
  - inspiring music, poetry or art
  - chocolate
  - a delicious meal or a glass of wine
  - a visit from a much loved pet
  - a hug from those who matter
  - a walk in the gardens in the sunshine
  - a gift of flowers, a letter or a visit from a friend
  - a beautiful view and a glorious sunset

Is this contemporary spirituality?

The only time I felt really spiritual was when I escaped throughout the church doors into the natural world again, where I sometimes genuinely felt inexplicable feelings of awe and wonder, when say the light on a leaf would astonish me. I would experience that ineffable feeling that wells up within us, between a breath and a heartbeat, that momentarily arrests us with a sense of something far greater than ourselves, but is gone by the time we reflect on it. That moment which – to adapt Dylan Thomas: ...makes us laugh, cry, prickle, be silent, makes your toenails twinkle, makes you want to do this or that, or nothing.

It seemed that to trust in this intuitive response might not be belief – in the way that it is taught by organised religion – but the willing suspension of disbelief. A willingness to be transported to a state of uncertainty when an indefinable experience can work through our hearts in a mysterious way that leads to love and compassion and humility and seems to be to me the key to our humanity. (Stubbs, 2000)

This highly articulate quotation describing one woman's perception of a spiritual experience is one that I am sure many of us can relate to. It is an excellent summary of the nature of contemporary spirituality.

The issue of whether a nurse should ever disclose a personal faith to a patient, however well meaning, has become the subject of a number of high-profile media stories and has caused intense debate. Whatever the rights and wrongs of individual cases, the position of the Nursing and Midwifery Council on this subject is not so clear-cut. Statements in the code (NMC, 2008) talk about recognising equality and diversity, using listening skills, non-discriminatory practice and dignity. Collectively they point towards a view that individual nurses should be guided by the person's agenda throughout, offer impartial advice where requested and use the explicit skills mentioned in this chapter and in Chapter 7 on communication to facilitate a conversation that explores *their* meaning of *their* life's events. In other words, personal disclosure is not recommended, because of the potential for such information to compromise the professional neutrality of the nurse and influence the patient towards a particular viewpoint.

Where to now?

Support for the development of spiritual care services in all areas where people die has in recent years come from government level. The 2004 Supportive and Palliative Care Guidance document, which is shaping all palliative care service development in the UK has a specific chapter dedicated to this subject area (NICE, 2004). Recommendations include:

- Improving access to spiritual support according to need
- Those delivering such support to be educated to agreed level
- Integrating spiritual support into multidisciplinary teams
- The recognition that such care is the responsibility of the whole team

Since 2004, therefore, there has been a national imperative to fund and integrate the spiritual element of care in all care environments and to make sure that it is not confined solely to formal religion. You will notice that the recommendations talk about the whole team. In order to further strengthen this, the publication of the Government's End of Life Care Strategy (DoH, 2008), which reports on the five-year development of integrated care plans in palliative care, has a strong emphasis on the need for spiritual care assessment and support for both patient and family.

Conclusion

No longer can this often misunderstood and ignored facet of care be conveniently ignored in clinical practice or abrogated into the hands of another perceived expert. There is a clear duty inherent within all nursing practice to address such needs.

All nurses can recall the sense of guilt they felt when they stopped to talk with a patient in the middle of a busy shift when it seemed that a thousand jobs needed doing. Forget the guilt, and next time stay with that patient a little longer, because it might just be that brief encounter and the care you demonstrate in those moments that really makes the difference. Time is always a factor cited by nurses as a reason for not being able to address spiritual needs, but it need not necessarily be dependent on time. Just like the concept of palliative care, as discussed in Chapter 1, it is a way of thinking and an attitude of mind that communicates respect, love and understanding to another.

References

Becker, R. (2001) Spiritual care on the rocks. *European Journal of Palliative Care*, **8**(4), 136.

Catterall, R., Cox, M., Greet, B., Sankey, J. and Griffiths, G. (1998) The assessment and audit of spiritual care. *International Journal Of Palliative Nursing*, **4**(4), 162–8.

Department of Health (2008) *End of Life Care Strategy. Promoting High Quality Care for all Adults at the End of Life*. DoH, London.

Granstrom, S. (1985) Spiritual nursing care for oncology patients. *Topics In Clinical Nursing*, **7**(1), 35–45.

Kemp, C. E. (1994) Spiritual care in terminal illness. *Journal of Hospice and Palliative Care*, **11**(6), 31–6.

Kristeller, J. L., Sheedy, Z. X. and Schilling, R. F. (1999) I would, if 1 could: how oncologists and oncology nurses address spiritual distress in cancer patients. *Psycho-oncology*, **8**, 451–8.

McSherry, W. and Draper, P. (1997) The spiritual dimension: why the absence within nursing curricula? *Nurse Education Today*, **17**, 413–17.

McSherry, W. (2007) *Meaning of Spirituality and Spiritual Care Within Nursing and Health Care Practice*, Quay Books, London.

Milne, A. A. (1992) *The Pooh Book of Quotations*, p. 41. Methuen Children's Books, London.

National Institute for Clinical Excellence (2004) Spiritual support services. In: *Improving Supportive and Palliative Care for Adults with Cancer: The Manual*, Ch. 7. NICE, London.

Ross, L. A. (1994) Spiritual aspects of nursing. *Journal of Advanced Nursing*, **19**(3), 439–47.

Ross, L. A. (1996) Teaching spiritual care to nurses. *Nurse Education Today*, **16**, 38–43.

Stubbs, I. (2000) We need solace to help use brave the secret undiscovered road ahead. *Daily Telegraph*, Weekend Supplement, 16 December.

💻 Useful websites

Beliefnet
http://www.beliefnet.com/

National Cancer Institute
http://www.cancer.gov/cancertopics/pdq/supportivecare/spirituality/Health-Professional/page1

Global Oneness
http://www.experiencefestival.com/spiritual_beliefs

Marie Curie Cancer Care
http://www.mariecurie.org.uk/forhealthcareprofessionals/spiritualandreligiouscare/

Cancer Care – Reading Room
http://www.cancercare.org/reading_room/ask/archive/spirituality-archive.php

The Freethinker
http://freethinker.co.uk/

Spirituality and Health
http://www.spiritualityhealth.com/newsh/items/home/item_216.html

Spirituality Assessment Tools
http://www.chcr.brown.edu/pcoc/Spirit.htm#Spiritual%20Well-Being%20Scale

Spirituality
http://www.spirituality.com/

📋 Chapter links to the Nursing and Midwifery Council Standards of Conduct, Performance and Ethics for Nurses and Midwives (2008)

Section 1: Make the care of people your first concern, treating them as individuals and respecting their dignity

Treat people as individuals
- You must treat people as individuals and respect their dignity
- You must not discriminate in any way against those in your care

■ You must treat people kindly and considerately
■ You must act as an advocate for those in your care, helping them to access relevant health and social care, information and support

Collaborate with those in your care
■ You must listen to the people in your care and respond to their concerns and preferences
■ You must make arrangements to meet people's language and communication needs
■ You must share with people, in a way they can understand, the information they want or need to know about their health

Work effectively as part of a team
■ You must make a referral to another practitioner when it is in the best interests of someone in your care

Act with integrity
■ You must demonstrate a personal and professional commitment to equality and diversity

☑ Self-assessment test

1. Spiritual care can best be described as:
    A How a person perceives heaven and hell
    B How someone ascribes meaning to their relationships with others, self and their life
    C A belief in the origins of the universe
    D The practice of religious rituals and religions

2. Tom is a 40-year-old plain-speaking electrician with no formal religious beliefs and regards such things as a 'load of rubbish'. He now has terminal cancer and asks you 'Do you really think their might be life after death?'. The most appropriate response would be:
    A Stay with him and explore his thoughts and feelings about his illness and his life
    B Tell him that you also believe such ideas to be 'a load of rubbish'
    C Suggest that if he wants to talk about such things in more detail you will give the chaplain a call
    D Disclose your own faith to him and reassure him that there is indeed life after death

3. Spiritual needs are often cited as universal to all humanity. Such needs can include:
   A Achieving career and financial success
   B Following a vocation
   C Keeping a sense of identity, value and worth in life
   D Going on adventurous holidays to broaden your knowledge of other cultures

4. Religious needs can best be described as:
   A Reading holy texts and learning about a faith
   B Visiting holy places
   C Participating in individual or corporate worship
   D All of the above

5. Nurses find dealing with spiritual needs difficult because:
   A Not many have a faith from which to draw guidance
   B It is seen as a private issue that should not be discussed
   C They lack the confidence to stay with and listen to a person asking profound, rhetorical questions
   D It is seen as only the job of the chaplain

CHAPTER 13

Palliative care emergencies

 Fifty, fit as a fiddle and a committed family man. He complains of backache, goes to A&E and is admitted to the ward. Three days later he can no longer walk and his life is filled with hoists, slings, catheters, morphine and hospital beds. He's paralysed from the waist down as the cancer spreads and pushes on his spinal cord, and his face is full of fear, worry and loss. It's all too much to comprehend.

Learning outcomes

After reading this chapter and completing the reflective activities the learner will be able to:

- Describe a range of palliative care emergencies that require intervention to relieve suffering
- Explain a number of strategies to help in such emergencies
- Understand better the true significance of quality of life for those facing terminal illness

Introduction

For some nurses the very idea that there could be life-threatening emergencies in those that are dying that require immediate actions to relieve suffering is a contradiction in itself. Indeed, the philosophy of palliative care is centred around the central notion of allowing someone to live until they die. To intervene in a situation that threatens to end life, thereby maintaining life, would at first glance seem to challenge this precept, yet it is the relief of suffering that is the primary objective, not the prolongation of life. With this in mind there is no contradiction and it is the duty of all nurses to be aware of the small number of emergencies that may occur and what can be done to help alleviate the distress encountered.

It is worth emphasising that emergencies in palliative care are rare, yet when they do occur they can have dramatic consequences for the patient. Some symptoms can be actively managed to significantly improve life quality, whilst others involve conservative management only to allow for as peaceful a death as possible. Whilst the primary prescription of the required medication is a medical duty nurses have a clear and important responsibility in this area. It is often nursing staff who first spot the rapid deterioration of the patient's condition and once the medical team have administered whatever course of action is appropriate it is the nursing team who then monitor and care for the person.

Ethical and professional questions

Before any major intervention is considered in a palliative emergency context there are a number of important questions that the whole team needs to ask of themselves, the patient (if possible) and the family.

- What does the patient want? Have they made an explicit written or verbal statement stating their preferences in an emergency (i.e. advance directive, do not resuscitate direction, or preferred place of care)?
- If no such preference is known or cannot be obtained what are the family's wishes?
- What is the specific problem?
- What are the chances of it being successfully reversed or managed to improve quality of life?

⏳ Reflective point

Any intervention needs to be weighed carefully for its potential benefits or harm. If no clear benefits can be seen to be achieved and the evidence available suggests that life quality will not improve or indeed potentially deteriorate then it is acceptable for comfort measures only to be used. That does not mean withdrawing care – it simply means that care adopts a conservative orientation towards essential comfort measures (see Chapter 14 for more details).

The primary emergencies reported in the current literature (Buckley, 2008) and experienced in clinical practice are:

- Spinal cord compression
- Hypercalcaemia
- Haemorrhage

- Superior vena cava obstruction
- Agitated terminal delirium

All these symptoms are synonymous with a cancer diagnosis and the empirical experience of management has arisen from the cancer arena. Whilst haemorrhage at the end of life can indeed be a feature of other diagnoses (chronic liver disease for example), the catastrophic nature of such haemorrhages via bleeding oesophageal varices frequently militates against any successful palliative measures.

Spinal cord compression

This is a condition associated with tumours metastasising around the spinal cord and occurs in approximately 3–5% of patients with cancer (Mallett and Dougherty, 2003). The primary cancers that can cause such metastases are breast, lung and prostate (Twycross and Wilcox, 2001). The signs of SCC (such as back pain around the lumbar region, motor deficits in the limbs and decreased strength) can present themselves several weeks before total compression occurs and it is beholden on nurses to look for these as indicators. Patients will often complain of not being able to lift previously easy household items and say they have pins and needles or numbness in their hands and feet, and sometimes urinary retention. There may also be a loss of coordination and they are unsteady on their feet. Taken individually such symptoms can simply be a complication of generalised weakness from cancer and bed rest, so can easily be missed. It is the bigger picture, built up over a period of time, that should sound alarm bells ringing and the only way to do this is to conduct regular assessment of the patient's neurological function.

When diagnosed, treatment needs to be prompt and success will depend on the overall condition and mobility of the patient. Treatment options include:

- Dexamethasone (a steroid to reduce inflammation around the tumour) and/or palliative radiotherapy to the tumour site. These are often done concurrently.
- Referral to the oncologist, who may be able to recommend either surgery (i.e. laminectomy to decompress the spinal cord), or in some cases a spinal block. This will reduce pain but will not increase mobility. (Twycross and Wilcox, 2001)

Nursing priorities

- Discussion with the patient of the options available
- Reassurance of thorough assessment and rapid treatment
- Explanation of the effects of the treatments of choice (i.e. the aim is to reduce pain and increase mobility)
- To anticipate anxiety during the treatment phase and offer realistic hope
- Monitor their neurological status and record as such
- Note changes in urinary and bowel function –sometimes catheterisation may eventually be necessary
- Monitor skin condition

Top priorities:

- Careful positioning of the patient in bed to stabilise the spine and reduce the potential for twisting and torsion
- Careful movement for bed bathing and positioning on a bed pan
- Check local manual handling procedures and uses aids where appropriate

Hypercalcaemia

This potential emergency is also associated with those patients who have tumours metastasising around the spinal cord and other bones in the body and is the commonest life-threatening metabolic disorder for those people with cancer. Those with myeloma and breast cancer have the highest incidence (Buckley, 2008).

As the word 'hypercalcaemia' suggests, it is an excess of calcium in the blood stream usually caused by tumour infiltration in the bone structure. It is definitively diagnosed by a blood test for serum calcium concentration, the normal levels being 2.7 mmol/litre. Symptoms are only difficult when the level reaches 2.9 mmol/litre or above. A level of 4.0 mmol/litre is usually fatal.

The presenting symptoms that can be observed include:

- Sudden incidence of confusion and disorientation
- Anorexia and vomiting
- Constipation
- Nausea
- Thirst and polyuria resulting dehydration
- Excessive fatigue

Many of these signs are common in people with cancer without hypercalcaemia. It is frequently the rapid change in mental state that first alerts the team and it is important that all nurses are aware of this. Treatment is thankfully simple and very effective in the majority of cases. The person's mental and physical condition can usually be restored to pre-hypercalcaemia levels within 48 hours, and often much sooner. Treatment options include:

- Correct dehydration via an intravenous infusion: 2 litres of saline over 24 hours is effective
- If serum calcium is 3.0 mmol/litres or over then biphosphonates given intravenously are the drug of choice – e.g. zoledronic acid, disodium pamidronate, sodium clodranate

Nursing priorities

- Discussion with the patient of the options available – where possible
- Reassure family of rapid treatment – they may be anxious at the sudden mental changes
- Monitoring of the infusion and care of the infusion site for signs of infection
- Explanation of the effects of the treatments of choice (i.e. the aim is to reduce the calcium level and to rehydrate the person)
- To anticipate anxiety and behavioural changes during the treatment phase

Haemorrhage

Problems with bleeding may be acute in nature, e.g. directly from a tumour site, arterial bleeds due to tumour invasion, or from associated local tissue trauma. Bleeding may also be more chronic in nature (e.g. from a fungating wound, peptic ulceration, or perhaps from anticoagulation therapy). NSAIDs (Non-Steroidal Anti-Inflammatory Drugs) can also cause bleeding.

Management of haemorrhage will depend on the site and nature of the bleed, but essentially it falls into two categories: acute and non-acute. The medical management of acute pain sometimes involves the prescription of intravenous or intramuscular midazolam (a sedative) and/or diamorphine (for the rapid relief of associated pain).

Nursing priorities – acute

- This can be extremely distressing for both the patient and the nurse supporting. Therefore it is essential that all areas have a clear policy to deal with this
- Stay with the person the whole time, offering compassionate, supportive presence and physical touch, e.g. holding hands – if this is acceptable
- Provide a constant presence at the bedside in the early stages
- Make sure the whole team are aware and relieve the supporting nurse after a certain agreed time
- Have dark-coloured towels available to soak up potentially large quantities of blood. The dark colour is more discreet.
- Ensure privacy around the bedside
- Reassure and support the family, who can become very distressed
- Debrief staff after the event

Nursing priorities – non- acute

- Discussion with the patient of the options available
- Reassurance of thorough assessment and rapid treatment
- Explanation of the effects of the treatments of choice (i.e. the aim is to reduce pain and bleeding and increase comfort)
- A review of all medications to rule out causative prescriptions
- Treat any aggravating infections with antibiotics
- Replacement of blood clotting factors where necessary. Vitamin B12 and plasma may help
- Wound management, including non-adherent dressings, or dressings to absorb exudates such as alginates or hydrocolloids
- Malodour – acceptable air freshening products, charcoal dressings
- Support the family throughout

Superior vena cava obstruction

The main causes of SVC occlusion are either extrinsic pressure on the vessel wall or direct invasion of the vessel wall by tumour infiltration. Most cases are due to a tumour within the mediastinum, of which up to 75% will be primary bronchial carcinoma (Fallon and Hanks, 2006). The presenting symptoms include:

- Breathlessness
- Headache and dizziness
- Neck and facial swelling
- Choking sensation
- Arm and trunk swelling
- There may also be dilated neck and collateral veins of the arms and chest
- Engorged conjunctivae with periorbital oedema

The most distressing symptom for the patient that requires immediate attention is dyspnoea and the sensation of drowning in fluids which is very frightening for the person. Direct management of this emergency is mostly medical in nature and includes high-dose corticosteroids such as dexamethasone, radiotherapy to the mediastinal lymph nodes and possibly surgery to insert a stent into the SVC to improve blood flow. Anxiety can be high, so the use of small doses of opioids, such as morphine 5 mg 4 hourly, can be useful.

Nursing priorities

- Discussion with the patient of the options available – where possible
- Explanation of the effects of the treatments of choice (i.e. the aim is to reduce the swelling around the vessel to improve breathing and general condition)
- Reassure family of rapid treatment – they may be anxious at the visual changes
- Monitoring of the effects of the giving of high dose steroids
- To anticipate anxiety and behavioural changes during the treatment phase and offer support and comfort via a constant presence at the bedside in the early stages

Agitated terminal delirium

In acute care and long stay settings, where experience of prescribing appropriate medication for dying patients close to the end of life is limited, the onset of delirium can be very difficult for the family and the caring team to manage. It does not represent a medical emergency in that the person's life is not threatened, but it does represent a very serious behavioural management issue that is frightening for the patient, the family witnessing it and indeed the nurses who have the primary responsibility to instigate care. Student nurses are often at the bedside when this phenomenon is present and have an active part in the overall care offered. The presenting symptoms include:

- Rambling incoherent speech
- Visual and auditory hallucinations
- Paranoid ideas
- Aggressive behaviour
- Constant restlessness

The causes of such confusion are many and it is worth noting them as it is often assumed that such episodes are simply a matter of cerebral hypoxia due to the normal dying process. Where there is an identifiable cause measures can be taken to alleviate the symptoms. Potential causes include:

- Prescribed drugs – opioids or antidepressants
- Infections – urinary, chest
- Severe constipation – especially in the elderly
- Metabolic reasons – hypercalcaemia, uraemia, hyponatraemia, hyper- or hypoglycaemia, or liver failure
- Alcohol or drug withdrawal
- Intracerebral tumours or strokes

Management of terminal delirium is by the prescription of drugs such as haloperidol 5 mg given subcutaneously or intravenously and if no effect no effect after 30 minutes then doubled to 10 mg. Midazolam, which is a sedative, is also a drug of choice for some doctors often in a dose of 10 mg subcutaneously. Some doctors may also prescribe chlorpromazine 50–100 mg intramuscularly every 4 hours, especially for the more florid hallucinatory symptoms. These doses are conservative and many medical practitioners will give considerably more depending on how the person responds. They can also be given via a syringe driver to ensure a continuous dosage over 12 or 24 hours.

Nursing priorities

- This can be extremely distressing for both the patient and the nurse supporting; therefore it is essential that all areas have a clear policy to deal with this
- Stay with the person, offering compassionate, supportive presence and physical touch, e.g. holding hands – if this is acceptable
- Provide a constant presence at the bedside until the medication takes effect and the situation calms

- There is a marked risk of the patient attempting to climb out of bed or injuring themselves on furniture around the bedside, so be careful to ensure that extraneous furniture is removed
- Cushions can be used around the bed to minimise movement
- Make sure the whole team are aware of what is happening and relieve the supporting nurse after a certain agreed time
- Ensure privacy around the bedside
- Reassure and support the family, who can become very distressed
- Debrief staff after the event

Conclusion

Nurses have a vital part to play in the overall care of the patient both during and after the medical management of palliative emergencies. The importance of this cannot be overemphasised, as in the rush to alleviate symptoms it is easy to lose sight of the patient's psychological, emotional and spiritual distress. In some cases this can be worse than the physical elements and nurses have a duty of care to address these important holistic needs. What must also not be forgotten are the needs of the nurses, who in dealing with intense emotive crises such as these will need support from colleagues, mentors and others to enable them to reflect and learn from the experiences.

 Reflective activity

Make sure that you have a record of the contact numbers and names of your local specialist palliative care team in your diary or notebook every time you go on duty. They will be able to advise junior or inexperienced staff as to the most appropriate course of action in the patient's best interest.

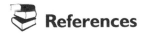 **References**

Buckley, J. (2008) Palliative emergencies. In: *Palliative Care: An Integrated Approach.* Wiley Blackwell, Chichester

Fallon, M. and Hanks, G. (eds.) (2006) *ABC of Palliative Care*, 2nd edn. Wiley Blackwell, London.

Mallett, J. and Dougherty, L. (eds.) (2003) *Manual of Clinical Nursing Procedures*, 5th edn, Ch. 38. Royal Marsden Hospital, Blackwell Publishing, Oxford.

Twycross, R. and Wilcox, A. (2001) *Symptom Management in Advanced Cancer*, 3rd edn. Oxford, Radcliffe Medical Press.

Recommended text:

Currow, D. and Clark, K. (2006) *Emergencies in Palliative and Supportive Care*. Oxford University Press, Oxford.

Useful websites

Palliative care drugs
http://www.palliativedrugs.com/

Downloadable factsheet on palliative emergencies
www.arthurrankhouse.nhs.uk/documents/.../Factsheet_16.pdf

Care Search – Palliative Care Knowledge Network
http://www.caresearch.com.au/caresearch/ProfessionalGroups/GPHome/
ManagingSymptoms/ManagingEmergencies/tabid/1154/Default.aspx

Chapter links to the Nursing and Midwifery Council Standards of Conduct, Performance and Ethics for Nurses and Midwives (2008)

Section 1: Make the care of people your first concern, treating them as individuals and respecting their dignity

Treat people as individuals
- You must treat people kindly and considerately
- You must act as an advocate for those in your care, helping them to access relevant health and social care, information and support

Collaborate with those in your care
- You must listen to the people in your care and respond to their concerns and preferences
- You must make arrangements to meet people's language and communication needs
- You must share with people, in a way they can understand, the information they want or need to know about their health

Ensure you gain consent
- You must ensure that you gain consent before you begin any treatment or care
- You must respect and support people's rights to accept or decline treatment and care
- You must uphold people's rights to be fully involved in decisions about their care
- You must be aware of the legislation regarding mental capacity, ensuring that people who lack capacity remain at the centre of decision making and are fully safeguarded
- You must be able to demonstrate that you have acted in someone's best interests if you have provided care in an emergency

Section 3: Provide a high standard of practice and care at all times

Use the best available evidence
- You must deliver care based on the best available evidence or best practice.

Keep clear and accurate records
- You must keep clear and accurate records of the discussions you have, the assessments you make, the treatment and medicines you give and how effective these have been
- You must complete records as soon as possible after an event has occurred
- You must ensure any entries you make in someone's paper records are clearly and legibly signed, dated and timed

☑ Self-assessment test

1. Which of the following statements about terminal delirium is true?
   A The drug treatment of choice is always an opioid analgesic
   B Family members should be asked to leave because their presence may increase the agitation
   C Placing the patient in a darkened room can help to calm matters
   D Providing a constant reassuring presence at the bedside can help support both the patient and family

2. The most appropriate treatment for hypercalcaemia is:
   A Correct dehydration by IV fluids and possibly bisphosphonates
   B Sedate the patient to relieve the anxiety
   C Give neuroleptics to address the confusion
   D Regular blood tests for serum calcium levels

3. Alfred has a large and fungating tumour on his neck that has started to bleed and is now pressing on his major blood vessels. He knows he does not have long to live. The nursing priorities are:

   A Make sure he has privacy around his bed

   B Keep dark coloured towels readily available

   C Review his medication to ensure good pain control and wound management to reduce both smell and exudates

   D All of the above

4. Which of these statements is relevant to the diagnosis of spinal cord compression?

   A It almost always of rapid onset

   B Success at treating it is excellent

   C Indicators are neurological and can appear slowly over some weeks

   D Permanent paralysis is inevitable

5. When considering the best way forward to manage any palliative emergency it is important that:

   A The family's wishes are paramount

   B The patient's expressed wishes are recorded and adhered to

   C The team are clearly in the best position to judge 'best interest'

   D We should always strive to maintain life

PART 3

Life closure skills

This part is concerned with the nursing skills, knowledge and behaviours which are crucial to the comfort, support and dignity of the patient and family as they perceive it when life is close to an end, and thereafter. The focus is on the diverse range of holistic skills which are needed to enhance quality of life and to help the patient and family exercise choices in care and come to terms with their loss.

CHAPTER 14

Essential comfort measures at the bedside

There she was, hidden nearly by the crisp white sheet pulled up to her nose. Two withered hands gripped tightly to the edge of the sheet. Two soft bright eyes appeared from the abyss looking at me. 'Got a minute nurse? Hold my hand please?', she said. I asked her 'Are you frightened?'. 'No' she replied, then silence. After about a minute she looked at me and said 'I had forgotten what life felt like'.

Learning outcomes

After reading this chapter and completing the reflective activities the learner will be able to:

- Reflect on the relevance and importance of quality care around the bedside at the end of life
- Select from a range of strategies to enhance quality of life from a holistic perspective
- Examine care priorities at the end of life in your current work area and identify both good practice and development opportunities

Introduction

This chapter is intended to provide the nurse with a checklist of what will be referred to as 'essential comfort measures'. This area of care has often been referred to as 'basic' care. The implication of which is that it involves unskilled tasks of low importance. Nothing could be further from the truth, and this unfortunate attitude is demonstrated when the practice of keeping the patient's body clean and well cared for and the surrounding environment conducive to dignity and privacy is carried out as a routine and functional chore where the humanity of care is lost in deference to the completion of the 'task'. The essential comfort measures that embody such care are of vital importance to the overall wellbeing of our patients and those around the bedside.

As stated in Chapter 2, such care has been described as 'sacred work', in which the carer enters into the intimate space of the patient and touches parts of the body that are usually private (Wolf, 1989). This is a highly privileged position that demands respect, a high degree of skill and sensitivity to individual need that is so essential when caring for the dying patient.

The list of activities offered is not intended to be prescriptive, or to offer any particular framework or philosophical model, but simply to highlight the wide range of care skills and behaviours that may be appropriate at this sensitive time.

Caring for the patient's body and immediate surroundings at the end of life is one of the most common areas of activity in any nurse's daily life. It is also the area that is most taken for granted in all healthcare practice, and the preservation of dignity has become central to government policy for the older person (DoH, 2006).

The NHS Plan (2000) reinforced to the nursing profession the importance of getting the essentials of care right and of improving the patients experience. As a direct result of this document the *Essence of Care* (DoH, 2001) was launched to help practitioners take a much more patient-focused and structured approach. This was developed into the *Essence of Care* (DoH, 2003), which is now well established and sets a range of benchmarks for standards in essential care and a toolkit for clinical areas to use to evaluate these standards. To complement these documents we also have the National Council for Palliative Care document (NCHSPCS, 2006) which examines care priorities at the end of life and more recently the publication of the *End of Life Care Strategy* (DoH, 2008). These are important documents as they move back to centre stage this area of care which has arguably been neglected in the past.

Privacy and dignity

■ Consider such elements as the protection of modesty, the availability of some personal space for the patient, and respect for personal beliefs and identity (DoH, 2003).

Hair care

■ Establish how often the patient likes their hair washed and conditioned and use the patient's own shampoo and conditioner where possible.

- Combs, and brushes should be kept clean, and the hair blow dried preferably.
- Always make sure that the patient's hair is parted on the correct side and the trimming of beards and moustaches is done in accordance with the style the patient is used to.
- Don't forget that excess hair protruding from the nose and ear may also need trimming, particularly with men.
- Use dry shampoo where appropriate.

Eye care

- Check to see if the person wears spectacles or contact lenses, either routinely or for reading, and make sure these are clean and accessible.
- Observe for signs of infection such as redness around the eye or excessive discharge, and if present report this to the senior nurse on duty.

Mouth care

- Often forgotten in the busy environment of an acute ward, but vital to patient comfort.
- Check the mouth regularly for cleanliness and signs of infection and clean the teeth daily with the patient's preferred toothpaste and/or denture cleaner.
- Offer proprietary mouthwashes if they are available and desired or crushed ice if appropriate.
- Where the patient is immobile conduct an assessment of the mouth daily, and use a recognised proprietary product to regularly moisten the lips, or a lip salve stick if the patient prefers.
- Pineapple chunks can be used to moisten the mouth. These will also assist in cleansing the mouth due to the enzymes within the pineapple juice.

Ear care

- Use cleansing cotton buds gently around the visible area of the ear, taking great care not to put them too far inside the aural canal.
- Observe for ear wax build-up and seek advice about the use of use wax softener where needed.

- If the patient's ears need syringing then seek the advice of the person in charge, who will make arrangements for this procedure to be performed.
- Be aware that patients of all ages may have a recognised hearing deficit and therefore may wear a hearing aid as a matter of daily routine. This should be recognised on admission and all staff informed as such. Anecdotal stories abound of patients being labelled as confused in their responses to requests, when in fact they may have a hearing deficit and be either unable to tell someone or perhaps too proud.

Nose care

- Nasal congestion is uncomfortable and can impede respiration.
- Check the nose daily and if appropriate clean with cotton buds and have soft tissues or handkerchiefs available.

Nail care

- Many healthcare trusts today forbid nurses trimming and shaping of nails as part of routine care. The rationale behind this is that there is a risk of causing damage to the skin and therefore a possible infection risk.
- Always check the policies and procedure manuals in your locality first before attempting such care.
- This does not, however, preclude the nurse from observing for infections, such as athlete's foot. Where present, request referral to a chiropodist, especially if there are visible malformations such as corns, bunions or dry split skin which can be both painful and impede mobility.

Pressure area care

- Use a recognised tool to assess pressure area risk and review this assessment regularly, depending on the patient's condition
- Monitor any aids currently in use. Pressure-relieving mattresses will help minimise the risk of skin breakdown, but does not take away the need for careful repositioning. The patient needs to be kept clean and dry at all times.
- Careful positioning will help avoid pressure sores and minimise pain from stiff, uncomfortable joints.

Skin care

- Washing the patient and applying moisturising lotion will avoid dry skin. Gentle massage of the hands or feet using either moisturising lotion or dilute aromatherapy oils will aid relaxation and give comfort.
- Massage is one of the simplest and most therapeutic forms of touch a nurse can ever use with a patient. Contrary to popular myth it is not necessary to attend a course or be formally qualified to use gentle massage on the hands and feet as long as simple safety precautions are observed.
  - Firstly establish that this is acceptable to the patient; some cultures may find it offensive and there may be gender issues to consider.
  - Observe the hands and/or feet carefully to establish that there are no open cuts or abrasions, arthritic or swollen joints, or lesions or tumours visible. If any of these are present then clearly massage is contraindicated.
  - Also ask the patient or check the case notes to see if the person has any known skin allergies that may contraindicate the use of some products.
  - Find out what is available in your locality to use for massage and what the patient prefers in terms of hand creams, or perhaps aromatherapy oils. It is not necessary to use expensive products, and simple unperfumed moisturiser is perfectly adequate.
  - The benefit of such massage is entirely qualitative in the time and personal attention given to the person as much as the element of touch and relaxation.

Odours

- Strong smells around a bedside are both embarrassing for the patient and family and avoidable in most cases. They can come from a variety of sources such as body odour, urine, faeces, stale food in lockers, or wounds. How you deal with these smells will therefore depend on the source, so it is important to be both sensitive and discrete.
- Be aware that junior staff may not have experienced such smells before, so it is good practice to warn them of such before exposure. This can save the potentially embarrassing and stigmatising reactions that may occur otherwise.
  - Spray deodorisers that are so readily available in most clinical areas should be used with caution and away from the immediate bedside. The fine mist they give off can cause allergic sneezing reactions and increase restlessness. They also only serve to mask odours for a short time period.

- – Simple aromatherapy oils are very effective and cheap and easy to obtain.
- – Use relevant charcoal infused dressings to absorb odours from wounds.
- – Fungating wounds sometimes need to be treated with metronidazole.
- ■ Manuka honey dressings are very effective at absorbing odours, are cheap to purchase, and can be used on any kind of wound.

Bodily hygiene

- ■ Whilst the patient is capable regular baths or showers should be given as suits the patient's choice.
- ■ Much good care and conversation can take place in the privacy of a bathroom, where a nurse's listening and attending skills can be used to the maximum to facilitate the expression of fears, doubts and worries.
- ■ If the patient is close to death then full bed baths are intrusive and inappropriate at such a sensitive time so establish when to and when not to.

Wound care

- ■ Make sure that all dressings are secure and there is a regular assessment of wound condition.
- ■ If the patient is in pain from the wound then consider appropriate analgesia to relieve pain in the longer term and some prophylactic analgesia 20–30 minutes before the dressing is changed.
- ■ When the person is close to death the priority is to prevent leakage of fluids, so consider changing the dressing to a waterproof one.

Environmental issues

- ■ Consider where the bed is placed. It is common practice to use a side room for the terminally ill if available and where this is an active choice for patient and family this is appropriate. Some patients prefer to be in a bay area out of choice, however, because they are reassured by the more immediate staff presence.
- ■ Maximise natural lighting around the patient's bedside where possible. It is well known that a person's visual acuity deteriorates as they approach death, therefore the temptation to dim the lights should be avoided.
- ■ Try to avoid unnecessary clutter on and around the bed and make sure there is good ventilation and warmth throughout the day and night time.

- Fans can be useful in hot weather, but be careful not to create a continuous draft around the head of the person.
- Some noise is unavoidable such as the hum of the motor in a pressure-relieving mattress or the bleeping of medical equipment; however, efforts should be made to minimise such intrusions.
- Natural flowers or plants nearby can be much appreciated, but check first that the patient has no known allergies and that such plants do not intrude on the bed space too closely.

Activities

- Boredom is a big yet unacknowledged issue in healthcare environments, so it is important for the patient to have a range of activities to engage in if they so wish.
- Consider such simple things as a daily newspaper, journal, games, books, magazines and a pack of cards.
- Electronic entertainment is available in compact form now around the bedside with portable DVD players, laptops, music players and of course the television.
- In some areas games consoles may be available. These are not only with useful young people; adults can get a lot of enjoyment from them, especially the handheld variety which now have many more adult-oriented programs available.

Diet/nutrition

- The key things to remember here are small regular meals, high in calories to boost energy, and well presented.
- Assessment of nutritional likes and dislikes should be made and meals should be modified to suit the patient's wishes, with liberal interpretations of diabetic needs.
- If feeding is needed then extra time should be allowed for this important and often neglected function.

Belongings

- Making a patient's bed space personal to them is psychologically very important in any caring environment away from the home.

■ Encourage the use of photos, personal clothes and jewellery, make-up and personal toiletries.

Visits

■ Find out from the patient who is important in their life and do not always assume that it is the immediate family.
■ Make sure access is granted to these people and that the rest of the caring team know.
■ Be aware that the patient may tire easily with too many people around the bedside, so be their advocate when necessary to limit time.
■ Find out what the visiting policy is in your area and remember issues such as refreshments for the family and chairs around the bed.
■ Consider open visiting if the family has to travel a long distance and the patient is close to death.
■ The key element is to remain discreetly in the background, but available.

Pets as visitors

■ There is an increasing body of evidence that where pets are allowed to visit the person it is good for their mood and general wellbeing (Geisler, 2004).
■ Such contact increases self-esteem, helps the patient maintain what for them could be a very important relationship with their pet and reinforces a sense of normality.
■ There is rarely a direct policy forbidding such visits and it is usually left to the discretion of the person in charge. Always discuss this with the team first.
■ Find out beforehand who will bring the animal and keep control of it. Clearly any potential behavioural or house training issues need to be considered before a decision is made.
■ Also establish if any of the nearby patients are allergic to the animal itself. It is not unknown for some people to be allergic to either cats or dogs.
■ Once these simple precautions are observed most clinical areas are now happy to accommodate short visits and the other patients often enjoy observing the pet.
■ Consider contacting the local Pets as Therapy representative (see website link at the end of this chapter), who can arrange for an approved visitor to bring in their pets. This is a national charity which carefully screens all animals and owners prior to allowing them to visit any clinical area.

Cosmetics

- Looking and feeling good in how we present ourselves to the world is part of normal daily life for both men and women. The use of cosmetic products, such as perfume, deodorant, after shave and moisturisers, eye make-up and hair products is part of this.
- Find out what the patient prefers and be prepared to help them apply the product if necessary.

Sleep and rest

- Clinical areas are of necessity busy places, so make sure that there are quiet periods for the patient during the day; reduce intrusive noise (e.g. TV, radio, medication trolley).
- At night time consider alternatives to proprietary sleep-inducing agents (e.g. Horlicks, Ovaltine, small amounts of alcohol and maybe ear plugs).

Mobility

- Passive limb exercises for bed-bound patients are part of the nursing role, but consider also assessment by a physiotherapist where necessary.
- Pain should be well controlled before embarking on any such exertions.
- Shoes should be well fitting and any aids for walking readily available. Correct positioning of the patient in a chair or bed is crucial to comfort.

Bowel care

- Be aware that all opioids can cause constipation; therefore a laxative should be prescribed concurrently.
- Laxatives that act as both bowel stimulants and softeners are often the most effective choice.
- Consider intervention every third day if the bowels have not opened. However, if death is imminent mild constipation is not an issue and any such intrusion is neither comfortable nor desirable. Dignity is everything at this juncture.

Elimination

- If diuretics are prescribed establish the timing of this medication.
- If a catheter is *in situ* then check for infections and blockages and observe the colour and consistency of the urine.
- If the patient has specifically requested that a catheter not be inserted when they become incapable then this wish should be respected.

Futile medications

- When the patient is close to death a regular review of the total regime is crucial.
- The whole care team should ask themselves whether intravenous and subcutaneous infusions, and/or total parenteral feeding are useful and appropriate.
- The decision to withdraw such treatment is ethically, morally and legally defensible if the team agrees that it is in the patient's best interest. The family's views should be listened too and acknowledged, but are secondary in this instance.

Routine observations

- It is not necessary to record temperature, pulse respirations or blood pressure on a patient who is clearly close to death, except where instructed for clear medical reasons – for example when a procedure such as blood transfusion is in progress.
- It can be useful to monitor the pulse occasionally when the person is close to death. Increased speed and reduced strength of the pulse from what has been the norm is a sign that the heart is endeavouring to draw in as much oxygen as possible when all the bodily systems around it are beginning to close down.
- Where family are away from a bedside for a break or sleeping close by it can sometimes provide staff with an indicator that death may be imminent, thereby allowing a brief but indeterminate time period for the family to gather or to prepare themselves for the coming event. It must be stressed that this is not an exact science and is not evidence-based, but is founded on anecdotal experience.

Reflective activity

Take this list and compare the documentation in use in your locality against the essential comfort measures discussed in this chapter. If you have the Liverpool Care Pathway or a local adaptation of this tool in use then you will find that most of these elements will already be included within your documentation. Some, however, will not be.

If you do not yet use these tools your comparison may well highlight a number of areas where care could be improved.

Essential comfort measures	Your clinical area
Privacy and dignity	
Hair care	
Eye care	
Mouth care	
Ear care	
Nose care	
Nail care	
Pressure area care	
Massage	
Odours	
Bodily hygiene	
Wound care	
Environmental Issues	
Activities	
Diet/nutrition	
Belongings	
Visits	
Pets	
Cosmetics	
Sleep and rest	
Mobility	
Bowel care	
Elimination	
Futile medications	
Routine observation	

Conclusion

The range of comfort measures cited within this chapter is not exhaustive by any means, but it does cover the areas of direct relevance to patient care at the bedside. What can be achieved will be entirely dependent on the facilities available and the prevailing staffing levels. In the real world of clinical practice there are always a thousand reasons that can be cited for not adhering to systematic good practice. I also know that if care is approached in a holistic and individualised manner using the tools available then time is rarely an issue. Our patients have a right to such high-quality attention to detail in the last days of their lives and we have a duty to provide it. Not only is such care at the core of good nursing practice, but the value of it as 'essential care' is at long last being emphasised once more.

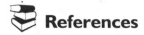 **References**

Department of Health (2000) *The NHS Plan: A Plan for Investment, A Plan for Reform.* The Stationery Office, London.

Department of Health (2001) *Essence of Care.* DoH, London.

Department of Health (2003) *Essence of Care: Patient Focused Benchmarks for Clinical Governance.* DoH, London.

Department of Health (2006) *Dignity in Care Campaign.* http://www.dh.gov.uk/en/SocialCare/Socialcarereform/Dignityincare/index.htm. Accessed: 18 February 2009.

Department of Health (2008) *End of Life Care Strategy. Promoting High Quality Care for all Adults at the End of Life.* DoH, London.

Geisler, A. M. (2004) Companion animals in palliative care: stories from the bedside. *American Journal of Hospital Palliative Care*, **21**, 285.

National Council for Hospices and Specialist Palliative Care Services (2006) *Changing Gear: Guidelines for Managing the Last Days of Life.* Clinical Guidelines Working Party, December 1997 (updated 2006).

Wolf, Z. R. (1989) Uncovering the hidden work of nursing. *Nursing Health Care*, **10**(8), 462–7.

 Useful websites

Essence of Care Programme
http://www.doh.gov.uk/essenceofcare

Pets as Therapy
http://www.petsastherapy.org

✒ Chapter links to the Nursing and Midwifery Council Standards of Conduct, Performance and Ethics for Nurses and Midwives (2008)

Section 1: Make the care of people your first concern, treating them as individuals and respecting their dignity

Treat people as individuals
- You must treat people as individuals and respect their dignity
- You must treat people kindly and considerately
- You must act as an advocate for those in your care, helping them to access relevant health and social care, information and support

Collaborate with those in your care
- You must listen to the people in your care and respond to their concerns and preferences
- You must support people in caring for themselves to improve and maintain their health
- You must recognise and respect the contribution that people make to their own care and wellbeing

Ensure you gain consent
- You must ensure that you gain consent before you begin any treatment or care
- You must respect and support people's rights to accept or decline treatment and care
- You must uphold people's rights to be fully involved in decisions about their care
- You must be aware of the legislation regarding mental capacity, ensuring that people who lack capacity remain at the centre of decision making and are fully safeguarded

Section 3: Provide a high standard of practice and care at all times

Use the best available evidence
- You must deliver care based on the best available evidence or best practice.
- You must ensure any advice you give is evidence based if you are suggesting healthcare products or services
- You must ensure that the use of complementary or alternative therapies is safe and in the best interests of those in your care

Keep your skills and knowledge up to date

- You must have the knowledge and skills for safe and effective practice when working without direct supervision
- You must recognise and work within the limits of your competence
- You must keep your knowledge and skills up to date throughout your working life
- You must take part in appropriate learning and practice activities that maintain and develop your competence and performance

Keep clear and accurate records

- You must keep clear and accurate records of the discussions you have, the assessments you make, the treatment and medicines you give and how effective these have been

☑ Self-assessment test

1. Delivering essential comfort measures to the patient at the end of life has been described as:
   A Mostly cleaning the person
   B Basic work
   C Sacred work
   D An important part of daily routine

2. You are asked to look after an elderly gentleman who is slipping in and out of consciousness. He is in a busy six-bedded bay. Which of these words best reflect the priority of care for this man?
   A Dignity and privacy, good mouth care, withdrawal of futile medications
   B Mobility, massage of limbs, pressure area care
   C Routine observations, good diet, plenty of fluids
   D Bowel care, sleep and rest, bodily hygiene

3. Whose direct responsibility is it to organise and deliver essential bedside care at the end of life?
   A The nurse in charge
   B The doctor overseeing the patient's care
   C The healthcare assistants and the students
   D All of the above

4. Essential comfort measures delivered with care and compassion will:
   A Extend the patient's life by a few hours or days
   B Directly enhance quality of life for the life that's left
   C Make the family feel better around the bedside
   D Conform to a designated pathway

5. The best combination of skills nurses need to deliver essential comfort measures includes:
   A Physical care skills and psychosocial care skills
   B Good teamwork and plenty of time
   C Attention to detail and a holistic patient-centred approach
   D Good organizational skills and the ability to delegate

CHAPTER 15

Multicultural needs at the end of life

🕊 *The apartment was small, cramped with possessions filling every available space. In the corner of the living room was a bed, facing the window. He turned and greeted us with a quizzical look; his mother meanwhile was busying herself finding drinks for her honoured guests. He was just 22 and the large cancerous tumour on his left thigh had spread to numerous parts of his body. Despite a regime of modern analgesia, it was clear that he was still in considerable pain. His expression, full of resignation and despair suggested to us that he knew both his diagnosis and prognosis and his mother confirmed as such. She was grateful for the support offered from the local palliative care team, because without it his pain had been unbearable and they spent time listening to her worries also. Family members had rallied round as is the tradition in that country and contributed what they could to help pay for the traditional medicines she dispensed to him throughout the day – medicines that gave some relief from the worst of the difficult symptoms (Becker, 2008).*

 Learning outcomes

After reading this chapter and completing the reflective activities the learner will be able to:

- Understand the broad concept of multicultural care as applied in a palliative care context
- Recognise a range of differing customs and traditions pertinent to different belief systems
- Personalise care of the individual to meet their cultural needs

Introduction

Cultural care is a diverse concept that embraces so much more than religion. As the story above illustrates, it is about social, economic, spiritual, and day-to-day coping within the norms, values, traditions and customs of the society in which you live.

The scene described could be in any one of dozens of developing countries around the world and characterises the many challenges palliative care services have to face day to day. It is in fact being played out in a suburb of Shanghai in southern China. This is one of the most modern cities in the world and is the economic hub of this vast country. The team looking after the young man mentioned above are one of 24 in major cities across China that are funded via the Li Ka Shing Foundation (LKS Foundation, 2008). Government support is moral rather than financial, a situation paralleled in many countries, but it's worth bearing in mind that 20 years ago such developments would have been impossible in the political climate of China.

Chinese attitudes to death and dying are quite unique, and whilst we in the west may find many aspects challenging there is much we can learn from them. When the Chinese talk of 'hospice' they do not mean a building, they talk of a philosophy and an approach that fits well with their traditional value system that has evolved over many thousands of years and embraces Confucianism, Taoism, Buddhism, Islam and even Christianity. They are therefore as multi-cultural in their attitudes and values as any western country.

It would be impossible within the boundaries of this short chapter to explore the differing palliative needs of the many citizens and their communities from around the world who populate the UK. Whilst the major religions of the world are declining in popularity in many western countries, with significantly fewer people having a personal faith to guide their lives, some of the less well known religions have grown in popularity. Conversely, a more secular approach to life founded in either an atheist or agnostic belief that there is not or may not be a god, has not necessarily created the problems of meaning at the end of life anticipated around the bedsides of the dying. Traditional cultural attitudes change and adapt to more widely held values no matter how controversial they may appear to some.

It is appropriate therefore that a diverse approach is adopted here to discuss the world's major and minor religions and their differing perspectives on dealing with death alongside some discussion on the needs of those without a formal faith.

⏳ Reflective point

Never assume adherence to any faith simply because of what may be written in a care plan stating the person's religion. Always ask the person, if possible, whether they follow the customs and rituals of their religion or not. Good nursing practice with those of another culture is based on the simple principle of individualised assessment and care of the person's expressed preferences. It is all too easy to fall into the trap of cultural stereotypes.

Christianity

Nursing considerations: close to the end of life

Christians believe that those baptised into the faith will share in Christ's resurrection and eternal life. If an adult requests baptism then this can be arranged through either the hospital chaplain or a minister of their choice.

- If an infant dies unbaptised the family may feel that the child has been excluded from the family of god and this can be distressing for them. In this instance baptism may be requested in an emergency for an infant, growing child or adult. Should a stillbirth occur then it is acceptable for a priest to conduct a naming and blessing ceremony soon after the birth.
- For those already baptised a priest may perform an anointing ceremony offering the 'sacrament'. They will use holy oil to make a sign of the cross on the forehead, chest and wrist of the dying person and prayers are offered.
- There are no dietary restrictions for the majority of denominations of Christianity and blood transfusions are acceptable.

Nursing considerations: after death

- Prayers may be said over the bedside or in the hospital chapel and last offices can be carried out according to normal practice.
- There are no moral restrictions on body donation along with organ usage for transplantation.

Islam

Nursing considerations: close to the end of life

- Those of the Muslim faith attach great importance to cleanliness, and hands, feet and mouth are always washed before prayer. In hospitals a shower is preferable to a bath where available.
- Muslim women will prefer to be seen by a female doctor and looked after by female nurses. Preservation of modesty is important.
- If a bedpan has to be used then have a bowl of water nearby for washing, as this is customary for both genders.
- The dying Muslim may wish to sit or lie facing Mecca, and moving the bed to make this happen will be greatly appreciated.
- Family members may wish to recite prayers around the bedside, so privacy is important. The Declaration of Faith (Al-Shahada) is said and if possible the dying person will respond 'I bear witness that there is no god but God and Muhammad is his messenger'.
- If no family member is available it is acceptable for any practising Muslim to give religious help if requested.
- Dietary restrictions during the month of Ramadan are usually suspended for those who are sick. Meat can be eaten as long as it has been slaughtered according to the Halal ritual which drains the meat of blood. Lamb, beef and chicken are eaten, but pork carrion and blood are forbidden. Fish and eggs are okay, but must be cooked where pork and other no Halal meat is cooked. Many families will bring these items in to a hospital or nursing home setting.

Nursing considerations: after death

- Where the attending doctor has issued a death certificate the body should be prepared according to the wishes of the family.
- The body should preferably not be touched by non-Muslims – therefore nurses should ask permission from the family and should always wear disposable gloves when closing the eyes and straightening the body.
- Body straightening should be done immediately after death, and this is done by flexing the elbows, shoulders, knees and hips first before straightening. This is done in the belief that the body will not stiffen.
- Do not wash the body, nor cut the nails or hair.
- Bandage the lower jaw to the head so that the mouth remains closed

- Turn the head to the right. This is so that the body can be buried with the face looking towards Mecca.
- Cover the whole body with a sheet.
- Burial should take place within 24 hours of death.
- Post mortems are forbidden unless ordered by the coroner, and organ donation is not usual. Body donation is forbidden.

 Reflective activity

Wherever you are on duty in whatever hospital, clinic, home or department make a point of taking a few moments to orient yourself to know which way is east. One day you may be asked to turn the bed of a deceased person to face that direction, and it is important to get it right.

Sikhism

Nursing considerations: close to the end of life

- Sikhs gain comfort from the reciting hymns from *Guru Grant Sahab* – the Sikh holy book. If they are too ill to do this then a relative or faith minister may do this.
- Sikh women will prefer to be seen by a female doctor and looked after by female nurses. Preservation of modesty is important.
- If possible, no turban should be removed from a man unless absolutely necessary. Likewise the 'kach' (breeches).
- If a bedpan has to be used then have a bowl of water nearby for washing, as this is customary for both genders.
- Many Sikhs are vegetarians and don't eat eggs or fish. Beef is forbidden, but some Sikhs will eat other meats.
- Blood transfusions are permitted.

Nursing considerations: after death

- In Sikh tradition the family are responsible for all ceremonies and rites connected with the body and many will want to wash and lay out the body themselves. However many are happy to let health workers conduct last offices. Consultation is the key.
- Do not cut any hair on the body as this is considered sacred.

- The face may be cleaned and the eyes and mouth closed.
- Limbs should be straightened and covered with a plain white sheet with no religious emblems.
- There are no objections to organ donation or post mortem examination.

Judaism

Nursing considerations: close to the end of life

- Orthodox Jews will wish for their body to remain covered for reasons of modesty, the women particularly so.
- The Sabbath (Friday) is observed by no travel or switching on of electric lights or appliances. Bedside lights and music systems can be turned on by others though. Bear this in mind.
- Some orthodox women will wear a wig, which should be kept in place, and possibly a head scarf. There is no restriction on care from both genders, but for Jewish women attendance by a woman is preferable.
- Only 'kosher' food is acceptable and the family will often bring in much of this. Milk and meat are not eaten at the same meal and pork and rabbit meat are forbidden. Fish must have fins and scales and shellfish is forbidden. A vegetarian diet is acceptable if no kosher food is available.
- Special psalms may be recited around the bedside (Psalm 23 and the Shema).

Nursing considerations: after death

- The body should be covered by a sheet and left untouched.
- The family usually take charge of body preparation after death, and the eyes may be closed and the limbs straightened by the children of the deceased.
- The family will contact the synagogue and the rituals necessary will be put in place.
- There is no objection in principle to organ donation as long as death is definitely established.
- Post mortems are not usual unless ordered by the coroner, and body donation is forbidden.
- Burial should take place within 24 hours of death.

Buddhism

Nursing considerations: close to the end of life

- It is the state of mind that is important for a Buddhist and time for meditation and peace is essential.
- There are no special requirements for Buddhists being looked after in a hospital or nursing home setting.
- Many Buddhists are vegetarian – always check this with the person.
- There are no objections to blood transfusions.

Nursing considerations: after death

- There are no formal rituals that need to be followed, so normal hospital practice for last offices is acceptable.
- The most important aspect is that the relevant Buddhist minister is informed as soon as possible.
- There are no objections to organ donation or post mortem examination.

Hinduism

Nursing considerations: close to the end of life

- Hindus will get comfort from readings and hymns taken from the Hindu holy book, the *Bhagavad Gita*. Family usually organise this, but if they are not available then contact the nearest Hindu minister.
- Holy rites may be requested and the Hindu minister can perform these. A dying Hindu should be given water from the Ganges and the sacred 'tulsi' leaf placed in the mouth by the family.
- Hindus prefer to die at home rather than hospital, so consultation with the family is essential if the person needs to be in hospital.
- Most Hindus do not eat beef or veal, some will not eat pork and many are vegetarian, often avoiding eggs. Explanation of the contents of unfamiliar dishes is particularly appreciated. Fasting is an important feature of Hindu religious life.

- The left hand is not normally used for handling food whilst eating because of its use in toilet routines. Consequently, staff caring for the patient should avoid using their left hand unnecessarily.

Nursing considerations: after death

- The family will want to wash and prepare the body themselves, including closing the eyes and straightening the limbs. Where family are not available nursing staff should always wear disposable gloves.
- Jewellery and religious objects should not be removed from the body.
- The body should be wrapped in a plain sheet without religious emblems.
- Post mortems should only be conducted under coroners orders and burial is usually within 24 hours.

Bahai faith

Nursing considerations: close to the end of life

- There are no special requirements for the Bahai person being looked after in a hospital or nursing home setting and no special dietary requirements.
- Alcohol is not usual although may be acceptable if in approved medication.
- There is no formal objection to blood transfusion.

Nursing considerations: after death

- The body should be washed and wrapped in a shroud of cotton or silk. A special ring is placed on the finger. Prayers will be arranged by the family or the local Bahai community.
- There are no formal rituals that need to be followed, so normal hospital practice for last offices is acceptable.
- Organ donation and post mortems are also acceptable.

Jehovah's Witnesses

Nursing considerations: close to the end of life

■ They will want reassurances that blood will not be used against their wishes. Blood may be taken for pathology testing and all relevant modern medications are acceptable.
■ There are no formal rituals save the need for members of the witness community to visit.
■ No special dietary requirements are needed.

Nursing considerations: after death

■ There are no formal rituals that need to be followed, so normal hospital practice for last offices is acceptable
■ Areas such as organ donation and post mortem are matters for individual conscience.

Rastafarianism

Nursing considerations: close to the end of life

■ There are very few rituals for the dying save the use of prayer around the bedside.
■ Many Rastafarians dislike conventional medicine and use alternative medicine instead. Always check this with the person, where possible, or the family.
■ Dietary restrictions include no pork and sometimes fish. Many are vegetarian by choice.
■ Blood transfusion is discouraged, but may be acceptable if the person and family can be assured of no disease transmission.

Nursing considerations: after death

■ There are no formal rituals that need to be followed, so normal hospital practice for last offices is acceptable.

- Post mortem and organ donation is actively discouraged in the faith.
- As there is no formal structure to the faith there is no minister to call.

Zoroastrians

Nursing considerations: close to the end of life

- Hygiene is very important and a shower will be preferred to a bath; however, at the bedside a bowl of fresh water is acceptable.
- There are no formal dietary restrictions; however, some may not eat pork or beef and prefer a vegetarian diet. Always ask.
- There are no last rites before death, but prayers may be said.
- With the orthodox believer blood transfusions are not acceptable, so always establish this early on.

Nursing considerations: after death

- Routine last offices according to local procedure is acceptable, with the body being bathed prior to being dressed in white clothing
- Post mortems are forbidden unless enforced by the coroner, and body donation or organ donation is forbidden.

Mormons

Nursing considerations: close to the end of life

- There are no formal rituals for the dying, but support from the faith community is very important. Know how to contact these people.
- Most Mormons are health conscious and will avoid tea, coffee alcohol and tobacco. Vegetarianism is popular, but not specific to their beliefs.
- Blood transfusions are acceptable, as is all conventional medicine.
- Sometimes more orthodox Mormons will wear a special undergarment which is regarded as sacred. This may be laundered as necessary, but extra must be taken with it as it is considered private and symbolic.

Nursing considerations: after death

- Routine last offices according to local procedure are acceptable.
- The sacred garment if present must be placed on the body after it has been washed.
- Organ donation and post mortems are not forbidden and are a matter for individual conscience.

Humanists, atheists and agnostics

Nursing considerations: close to the end of life

- There are no formal rituals as these groups do not believe in a god or after-life, so normal hospital practice for last offices is acceptable.
- There are no dietary restrictions and issues such as blood transfusions are down to individual choice.
- Bear in mind that the hospital chaplain may not be welcome.

Nursing considerations: after death

- Routine last offices according to local procedure is acceptable
- Organ or body donation is a personal choice and post mortems are not objected to.

Pagans

Nursing considerations: close to the end of life

- Some Pagans may wish to have a small white candle and holder or a small figure of a goddess to hand for prayer and support.
- Dietary preferences include vegan, vegetarian and raw food diets.
- In the case of patients who are seriously ill or dying, it is important that the Pagan patient has the name and telephone number of their spiritual adviser so that he or she may attend.

Nursing considerations: after death

- There are no special rituals or observations in the case of death.
- Routine last offices according to local procedure are acceptable.

 Reflective activity

Find out what the principal faith communities are within your geographical area and make a note of these. Next time you are on duty check out the local policy and written information for contacting faith representatives and interpreters for non-English-speaking patients.

Communication issues in cross-cultural care are at the heart of both success and failure, so it's important to pay attention to these few simple rules:

- Listen carefully to the patient's story of their illness and circumstances and build a supportive, trusting relationship based on honesty and mutual respect.
- Make sure that what you say is clearly understood. A yes response does not necessarily mean that the patient understands what has been said. It may mean 'I heard you'. It is wise to ask the patient to repeat the information given back to you.
- Patients from certain cultures may defer to the authority of health providers in a paternalistic way and may be reluctant to ask questions about their care.
- In some cultures there is a reluctance to give eye contact with an individual perceived to be an authority figure and the patient may say 'no' to avoid embarrassment.
- Not everyone wants to know the details of their diagnosis, treatment and prognosis. This information will empower some; whilst others believe it causes hope to be lost and may hasten death.
- Complementary medicines are frequently used in healthcare alongside western medicines. Ask specific questions about their beliefs and practices concerning such medicines and therapies.
- Privacy, modesty and physical touch are highly sensitive areas of care and the norms for the patient should be established as early as possible.

Good practice guidelines

- Allow the patient to define her/his culture and community; ask the patient about the community's response to death and dying and whether they wish the community to be contacted.
- Determine the patient's value system by adding cultural questions to your assessment.
- In respecting patient dignity and self-determination, respect cultural differences even though you may not agree with them.
- Learn about the religious beliefs of the patient and how these beliefs influence the process of dying and death.
- If the person has no formal beliefs and is an expressed atheist, respect their position and discuss what their wishes are.
- If you do not speak the language of the patient, use trained interpreters. All NHS hospitals will have access to a range of interpreters for the main cultures within the area.
- Be aware that not all societies agree that patient autonomy, self-determination and truth telling are acceptable.

⌛ Reflective point

The Nursing and Midwifery Council requires all nurses to be neutral and non-judgemental in clinical practice, whilst respecting diversity. Occasionally, however, a nurse may be asked to self-disclose their own beliefs by the patient, or a nurse may chose to do so in the context of a conversation, because they believe it may help the person. There are instances where this has led to misinterpretation and offence, so be cautious about such disclosure. Only do so if requested and do not offer to engage with formal rituals, as this could be seen as exerting undue influence, however good the intent.

Conclusion

Awareness of multicultural needs in clinical practice depends very much on the population demographics of the area in which you work. If there are large established communities of several generations the healthcare services will be well geared up to address those needs. Conversely, in areas where such communities are rare communication issues and stereotypical ideas of what may be needed can be all too common. Immigration trends and movement from cities to rural areas in search of work in recent years have seen a radical shift in the diverse number of cultures around the UK and as such exposure to the needs of members of these groups has never been higher.

Cultural norms regarding acceptable treatment regimes, the expression of grief, the experience of pain and symptom control and truth telling vary hugely around the world and many people bring these differing values with them into healthcare and around the bedside when someone is dying. It will remain a challenge for all health professionals to learn about the differences, respect these values and beliefs and provide a good death as close as possible to the prevailing beliefs.

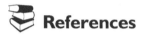

References

Becker, R. (2008) Attitudes to death and dying in China (editorial). *International Journal of Palliative Nursing*, **14**(10), 419.

Li Ka Shing Foundation (2008) http://www.lksf.org/eng/project/medical/hospice/main01.shtml. Accessed: 12 August 2008.

Recommended book:

Green, J. and Green M (2006) *Dealing with Death: A Handbook of Practices, Procedures and Law*. Jessica Kingsley, London.

 Useful websites

West Sussex Hospitals Chaplaincy Department
http://www.wsh.nhs.uk/chaplaincy/

Multicultural Palliative Care Guidlines. Palliative care Council of South Australia
http://www.pallcare.asn.au/mc/mccontents.html

Chapter links to the Nursing and Midwifery Council Standards of Conduct, Performance and Ethics for Nurses and Midwives (2008)

Section 1: Make the care of people your first concern, treating them as individuals and respecting their dignity

Treat people as individuals
- You must treat people as individuals and respect their dignity

- You must not discriminate in any way against those in your care
- You must treat people kindly and considerately
- You must act as an advocate for those in your care, helping them to access relevant health and social care, information and support

Collaborate with those in your care

- You must listen to the people in your care and respond to their concerns and preferences
- You must support people in caring for themselves to improve and maintain their health
- You must recognise and respect the contribution that people make to their own care and wellbeing
- You must make arrangements to meet people's language and communication needs
- You must share with people, in a way they can understand, the information they want or need to know about their health

Be open and honest, act with integrity and uphold the reputation of your profession

Act with integrity

- You must demonstrate a personal and professional commitment to equality and diversity
- You must adhere to the laws of the country in which you are practising

☑ Self-assessment test

1. Which of the following statements regarding multicultural care is most accurate?
   A It's all about attending to religious rituals and customs
   B It's best left to the experts in case we get it wrong and upset the patient and family
   C It's a diverse concept that brings in social values, customs and traditions
   D It's the same for all those of a particular faith

2. There are six main religions across the globe. They include:
   A Judaism, Mormons, Christian Science
   B Sikhism, Islam, Christianity
   C Rastafarians, Hindus, Buddhists
   D Bahai, Paganism, Jehovah's Witnesses

3. Which of the following is *not* part of good cross-cultural practice?
   A   Looking up faith traditions on the Internet and devising a care plan based on this
   B   Asking a person about their traditions, values and beliefs
   C   Finding out who the community leaders are in your area and knowing how to contact them if needed
   D   Respecting the traditions involving prayer and washing of the body after death

4. Nurses find it very challenging to deliver cross-cultural care at the end of life in hospitals because:
   A   The lack of privacy can make it difficult to address such needs
   B   If there are few other cultures in the area awareness of needs is low
   C   They are often reluctant to ask the patient and family what their wishes are
   D   All of the above

5. A patient says to you that they were brought up as a Catholic, but rejected the faith as an adult and now they are dying they don't know what to do. How do you respond?
   A   Tell them that you are a lapsed Catholic also and not to worry about it
   B   Sit with them, listen to their concerns and find out what their priorities are
   C   Give the priest a call and ask him to come and have a chat with him/ her
   D   Offer to pray with them at the bedside

CHAPTER 16

Care priorities in the last days of life

Connie was 82 with chronic renal failure and lung cancer. She had been married for 60 years and was her husband's principal carer. I found Connie in tears after lunch and she said 'All I want is to see my husband again, but I know he's too ill and in a wheelchair'. That evening, however, daughter and husband arrived and we took them to a sleeping Connie who woke up, grasped his hand and the two of them cried together. He looked at her longingly and said 'I wish I could hold you one more time'. It took about half an hour to organise, but we got him onto the bed beside her and left them in peace. The love in their eyes was a joy to see.

Learning outcomes

After reading this chapter and completing the reflective activities the learner will be able to:

- Describe the core knowledge, skills and attitudes required to meet the specific needs of patients in the terminal phase of life
- Support the needs of the family around the bedside of the dying person
- Reflect on current skills and knowledge levels in the care of the dying person in the last few days of their life.

Introduction

The story of Connie and her husband is an excellent example of how attention to the small details around the bedside to help meet a person's needs can make all the difference to their quality of life. It would have been easy to avoid making the effort to put the two of them together, particularly in our heavily regulated, health and safety-conscious work environments, but the team wisely planned it out carefully and made it happen for this devoted couple. Not only will Connie benefit from this small act of kindness, but her husband will carry with him the memories of his last intimate contact with his wife. As an illustration of exemplary, individualised care I can think of none better to introduce this chapter, which will focus on the holistic needs of those close to the end of their life.

Recent developments

The transition point between curative interventions designed to maximise health and those that are more palliative oriented is never easy to define with a patient in any care environment and represents one of the biggest challenges that all health professionals face in clinical practice. Government recommendations via the NICE *Supportive and Palliative Care Guidance* (NICE, 2004) quite rightly emphasise a partnership approach with patient, family and the multidisciplinary team working together to reach a decision that is in the patient's best interest.

Key messages from government policy documents (NICE, 2004)

- A good death is important for patients and families if this can be achieved with dignity, within place of choice and with symptoms well managed
- Sustaining the family during the illness and into bereavement reduces potential morbidity and lessens future demand upon the NHS and Social Services
- Good palliative care at the end of life, as well as being an appropriate compassionate response in a civilised society, also makes good economic sense

Anticipated outcomes of the End of Life Care Programme (DoH, 2008)

- Greater choice for patients in their place of care and place of death
- Decrease in the number of emergency admissions for patients who have expressed a wish to die at home
- Decrease in the number of patients transferred from a care home to a district general hospital in the last week of life
- Generalists skilled in the use of the models of care tools to improve end of life care

Once decisions regarding medical care have been made, however, it is nurses who have the primary responsibility for the delivery of such care, whether it is in a care home, acute ward, or the patient's home.

Within this scenario it can be equally as difficult to moderate that focus once again towards the more terminal phase of life. Those last few days and hours require a subtle but significant change in the approach to care, wherever that care takes place. This is where tools such as the Liverpool Care Pathway (Ellershaw and Wilkinson, 2003) come to the fore, because it is specifically designed to meet the needs of those dying in any environment. It provides multidisciplinary teams with documentation to underpin the comfort care that is given whilst a patient is receiving palliative care up to the point of their death. This documentation replaces all other notes, including both nursing and medical notes, and can act as a useful check list for the team to ensure that all the patient's and relatives' needs are fulfilled. The idea is that a seamless service is provided as clinical areas liaise with other agencies to smooth the care of the person towards a peaceful death. Essentially it is a template for patient centred best practice and can help to facilitate appropriate standards of record keeping in line with Nursing and Midwifery Council requirements (NMC, 2008).

Tools such as the LCP are, however, only as good as the user's competence and attitude towards the delivery of palliative care and at present it is far too early offer a full and objective opinion on its efficacy. Anecdotal evidence from around the UK would seem to indicate that where it has been successfully adapted to suit local needs it is beginning to make a difference. Uptake by healthcare trusts is optional, not mandatory, and therefore at present we have a patchwork across the country of mixed use at different levels (Help the Hospices, 2007). There is little doubt that these tools can be immensely helpful to nurses, but we must be cautious of using them in a reductionist manner as simply a tick box checklist where workload pressures are heavy. There is a very real danger, therefore, particularly in busy environments, of dehumanising the delivery of care to the lowest common denominator, with the holistic nursing focus getting lost along the way. It is for this reason therefore that no specific framework or tool is offered within the text. The focus is on good practice interventions to inform the reader of exactly how to achieve this orientation, which is so crucial to the quality of the short life that is left to those being cared for. Not all the good practice offered is suitable to all environments, but I am sure that you will find a wide range of options that are achievable within most settings.

The aims of the nursing management for care during the terminal phase are quite simple and entail:

■ The relief of distressing symptoms, fears and anxieties as far as possible
■ The provision of active support for informal caregivers

- Enabling patients to die in the place of their choosing, wherever possible and with a sense of dignity, as they perceive it
- Minimising the potential for a complex grief reaction associated with bereavement

The guiding principles underpinning care in the terminal phase are:

- Patient and family participation where possible
- A collaborative multidisciplinary approach by all relevant health professionals
- Use of appropriate medications tailored to each person given regularly to relieve and prevent symptoms
- Continued regular review of all care over the 24 hour period
- Access and early referral to specialist services for patient and family support if needed
- Support and acknowledge the uncertainty of how and when someone may actually die

The most commonly reported physical symptoms close to death include:

- Pain
- Dyspnoea
- Nausea/vomiting
- Agitation/restlessness
- Confusion
- Noisy breathing
- Urinary incontinence or retention
- Dry or sore mouth

Of these symptoms it is dyspnoea which is the most feared, not pain. It is the professional duty of the nurse to develop a good rapport with the patient and relatives so that such symptoms can be recognised quickly and dealt with accordingly. Whilst prescription of proprietary medication is the responsibility of the doctor, the bulk of care delivered thereafter is a nursing responsibility. It is useful, therefore, to look at the priorities of care from a holistic perspective.

Psychological care

This is perhaps one the most poorly addressed and undervalued areas of nursing assessment, yet for the patient it is often the one most closely associated with their suffering (Becker, 2007). A patient may fear that the pain they are experiencing could escalate into extreme agony and need reassurance that the regime prescribed will not let this happen. Some patients with extreme anxiety may even resist falling asleep for fear of stopping breathing in their sleep. The increasing dependency of the dying person, especially in a home environment, may contribute to the family feeling overwhelmed by the responsibilities they have to take on. There may also be strong opinions held by other family members or influential friends who have had a poor past experience of death that was neither peaceful nor dignified. Such strength of opinion can have a profound effect on a family's coping strategies.

Spiritual care

(See Chapter 12 for more detailed advice.)

This often misunderstood area is crucial to the wellbeing of the person and must not be ignored. We all have a need to find some meaning to difficult life events, in whatever context, and spiritual care needs to be viewed in this way. There are many ways of conceiving this, ranging from the more formal religious belief through to a more humanist or indeed atheist stance. What matters is that it is the nurse's duty to meet the patient where they are in their exploration of what dying means for them. Awareness of a person's cultural perceptions and belief systems about death and dying is therefore crucially important. Expect profound questions to be asked about death and meaning in life. This is normal, as it represents a search for meaning to the event unfolding before them. We may not feel able to give answers to more formal questions regarding religious faith, but we should know how to access the relevant faith minister, who can provide guidance and support. When someone become very weak there can sometimes be huge anxiety and distress associated with this, as there is a logical fear of losing control over events. There may also be unresolved conflict, or guilt between the family and the dying person. It is not unusual to feel tension around a bedside at times like this.

Physical care

Attending to the body and its functions is perhaps the most common and intimate duty a nurse can perform. Close to the end of life such care has a specific orientation that moves away from aggressive medical interventions and focuses on the need for comfort and quality of life.

Most of the duties implicit within this area have been discussed and are listed in the previous chapter under the heading of 'essential comfort measures'. Rather than repeat this bullet list it would be wise for you to refer to this list once more. There are, however, a number of other elements of good practice towards the end of life that fall under the auspices of physical care, described below.

The consciousness level

Most people who die an expected death slip in and out of consciousness over several days; therefore:

- Speak to the patient slowly and clearly, informing them of procedures before carrying them out. Even if the person appears unconscious it is good practice to speak to them as if they were conscious. This helps to maintain personhood and dignity.
- Speak to the relatives where appropriate and warn them of fluctuating consciousness and the possibility of disorientation and restlessness. Reassure them that is a normal part of the dying process and is not indicative of poor symptom control.
- Resist full body washes unless absolutely necessary in the hours immediately before death. Such washes are inappropriate in most cases.
- Be sure to keep the bedclothes loose.
- Stop oral fluids when consciousness fluctuates and be sure to say why this is important to the relatives (i.e. to prevent the person choking as the gag reflex is less effective).
- Have sips of water plus ice cubes available and maintain good mouth care.
- Intravenous and subcutaneous infusions should be taken down unless for a clear purpose (e.g. hypercalcaemia). This is a sensitive issue and medical staff should be challenged to justify the rationale behind maintaining intravenous or subcutaneous fluids close to death where this is the case. There is an increasing body of evidence that such invasive procedures can exacerbate dyspnoea and are of no benefit to the patient (Bavin, 2007). Do not fall into the trap of condoning such practice merely because it appeases the relatives, other nurses or medical staff.

Respiration

- Turn the patient from side to side at regular intervals to facilitate the drainage of secretions, but remember it is not advisable to move the patient when death is imminent.

- Leaving the patient on their back may cause the tongue to sag and result in a distressing snoring sound. Drugs such as hyoscine can help to dry excessive secretions and should be considered in such instances.
- Keep the nose and mouth scrupulously clean.
- Reassure the relatives that the shallow breathing they may be witnessing is not the person gasping for air but a normal aspect of dying.
- Sometimes the relatives may observe long pauses between breaths of up to 30 seconds or more (Cheyne–Stokes Breathing). If this begins to occur then reassure the relatives that this is a normal aspect of the dying process to alleviate their anxiety. Because of the intermittent nature of the breaths it can make determining the exact time of death quite difficult, therefore it is good practice that the nursing staff are close by during this period.

Cardiovascular system

- Monitor the patient's pulse discreetly and regularly. When death is imminent the pulse changes to become weaker and more rapid as the heart attempts to compensate for lack of oxygen.
- Encourage the relatives to check the patient's wrist pulse. This is easily done and can provide an early warning to the family of the impending death. If there are family nearby having a break then they can be contacted. NB: It must be stressed that this is not an exact science and is not evidence-based, but is founded on anecdotal experience.
- Change the bed linen and clothing as necessary.
- Light clothing and fresh air circulating is helpful.
- Do not put on extra blankets because the patient feels cold to the touch as this can cause restlessness.

The senses

- Try to maximise natural light wherever possible and to avoid the overuse of fluorescent strip lights, even though this may be difficult in a hospital situation.
- Keep the lights on in the patient's room. Visual acuity deteriorates as a normal part of dying and the patient may wish to be physically close to their family in order to see them clearly.
- Advise visitors to sit next to the patient and not at the end of the bed.
- Remove obtrusive furniture and equipment where possible to allow the family uncluttered access to the patient.

- Encourage conversation to be in normal tones and not whispers as the sense of hearing can remain acute right up to death.
- Keep all dressings clean, secure and waterproof to prevent any potential leakage of fluids.
- Use aromatherapy oils to promote a relaxing atmosphere and to help mask bad odours.
- Do not use spray deodorisers directly around the bedside as they can cause coughing and restlessness.

Caring for the relatives

As death approaches:

- Encourage them to touch, hold and talk to their loved one.
- Hearing is the last sense to be lost even if the person appears unresponsive.
- If several relatives are there, encourage some to take a break away from the bedside, but to remain close by and contactable.
- Be sure to keep them supplied with drinks and snacks if you can. They will be tired and inclined to ignore their own needs.
- Encourage them to do small things for their loved one (e.g. combing hair, cleaning the face).
- Explain the signs of impending death to the family where appropriate and with sensitivity. Remember that not all families require or request this; therefore it is a matter of careful judgement on the nurse's part whether this is the correct course of action.
- Reassure them that the death itself will be peaceful

At the moment of death and soon afterwards:

- Provide the family with time, space and privacy to stay with the deceased for as long as they wish.
- Encourage them to touch and hold the deceased, reassuring them that the body does not deteriorate quickly and remains warm to the touch for some time.
- If the person is from another culture it may be necessary to turn the bed to face the east. Establish first, via the family, whether this will be necessary or desired and also whether it is achievable within the clinical area.
- Encourage them to say goodbye and to express their feelings if they can. Open grief at this moment is both healthy and appropriate, but people often need permission from the professionals to express themselves.

- Remain discreetly in the background, but available if needed.
- Remember that they may be bewildered about what to do next. Therefore be sure to have the correct local procedure at hand, backed up with literature if possible.
- Don't forget that the eyes may not close at death so be prepared. Do not use any form of tape or coins to close the eyes as this may damage the delicate tissues. Damp cotton wool balls are the simplest and most effective solution and should be placed over the eyelids for approximately 2–5 minutes. This is usually enough time to train the muscles of the eyes to remain closed.

 Reflective activity

Next time you go on duty take a moment or two to orientate yourself so that you are aware of which direction is east and consider the practicalities of how you would move a bed to face that direction if it was requested.

Hospital-specific issues in terminal care

- Prescription of adequate doses of analgesia and other medications on a regular basis. Junior medical staff in particular need support and guidance.
- Appropriate verbal and written information for patients and relatives
- Recognition of the impact of death on the other patients in a ward. If a patient has been in a 4- or 6-bed bay for some time then they will have almost certainly formed relationships with those around them. It is both courteous and sensitive to the memory of the deceased to acknowledge the event to these people at an appropriate time.
- Careful handling of requests for post mortem.
- Support for relatives when they return to pick up patient's belongings after the death.
- Multi-professional decision when dealing with the transition to terminal care.
- Careful decision making regarding patient transfer to a hospice or specialist unit.
- Support for junior medical staff who often bear the brunt of breaking bad news as well as patient and family requests for information.
- Support in the clinical area for nursing staff who may have formed a continuing relationship with both patient and relatives.

Home-related issues in terminal care

It is rare for a nurse to be present in someone's home when a person dies, so it's important that the family are prepared for the event to come in a sensitive manner. It is a clear nursing duty to inform the family of the imminent signs of the terminal phase:

- Increasing tiredness/sleeping
- Confusion and/or restlessness
- Decreased intake of food and fluids
- Incontinence
- Diminished urine output
- 'Rattling' breathing
- Skin mottling

Many people have little or no personal experience of either seeing or dealing with a body, therefore it is useful to point out the signs of death itself:

- Patient stops breathing
- Patient cannot be roused by shaking or shouting
- Death is usually peaceful, not loud or violent
- Profound skin pallor develops within half an hour of death

It is also a nursing duty to instruct families about what to do after the event itself.

- Even though a death may be expected, a sense of panic can sometimes prevail when it occurs. It is important therefore that the family are told not to attempt to resuscitate or dial for an emergency ambulance (ambulance crews are obliged to begin resuscitation and take the body to the nearest hospital; this will be distressing for the family).
- Phone for the GP or appropriate local GP on-call service.
- Stress that there is no urgency about contacting an undertaker. If death occurs during the night this can be done the following day.
- Encourage the family to spend time with the body and to actively say goodbye.
- Inform the family about what reactions to expect (e.g. anger, crying, or even denial) and how to cope with extremes of emotional outburst or the reactions of children.
- Where children are present it is important that the family do not use phrases such as 'gone to sleep' as this can confuse them and can cause distress at night time.

Professional duties after a death

- Make sure that the key staff involved know what is happening and that the event is accurately recorded in the notes
- If organ donation has been requested beforehand then know how to contact the team concerned. The nurse in charge will most likely take on this responsibility.
- If death is within 24 hours of surgery, anaesthetic, or any invasive procedure then the Coroner needs to be informed. If this is the case it is important not to remove cannulae, tubes, or pack orifices before talking to the doctor concerned. If in doubt seek advice from a senior nurse.
- If body donation has been arranged then know where the university medical school concerned can be contacted. They will arrange to pick up the body from the nominated place.
- If a different culture is concerned then know where you can contact the appropriate community leader or minister, but only if this has been specifically requested. It's vital to find this out beforehand so don't assume that the family want this.
- Establish what rituals need to be observed before and after death with the body and who can be involved.
- Be clear about last offices procedure. This will not be discussed in this chapter as local procedures vary greatly around the country and are constantly being revised. Please refer to your local policy.
- Remember that as a junior staff member you may not have been involved in this before, so recognise your vulnerability here and seek support.
- Recognise the team's emotional needs at this time also and help arrange support.

✏ Reflective activity

What thoughts and feelings does the following story evoke? And what does it tell you about the dying process?

I asked myself where could she be? She seemed so very far away. Those big brown eyes stared up to the stars above. Her body, which never stopped moving when she was conscious, now lay still and fragile. Can she hear me? I thought. I really don't know. I leant over and pressed my lips to her cheek and whispered in her ear. There was no reply. I started to walk away tasting the salt from my tears. Then through a corner of my eye I saw a hand reach up and her long finger called me back. I know you do she replied, then returned to the place so very far away.

Conclusion

There is no greater privilege as a nurse than being part of the unique dynamics and care in the last few days and hours of someone's life. It is a very special honour and needs to be better recognised and valued within healthcare generally. The skills involved are truly holistic in nature and embody the best that nursing has to offer in terms of the science and art of practice. It will always remain an immense challenge in any environment simply because there is no right or wrong way to die, and the preferences of each person and how they interpret their dignity are unique to them. Our challenge is to attempt to understand that interpretation, meet them where they are on this journey, not pass judgement and help them in this unique event.

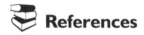 **References**

Becker, R. (2007) Psychosocial dimensions. In: *Palliative Nursing : Improving End of Life Care*, 2nd edn (eds. S. Kinghorn and S. Gaines). Baillière Tindall, Edinburgh.

Bavin, L. (2007) Artificial rehydration in palliative care: is it beneficial? *International Journal of Palliative Nursing*, **13**(9), 445–9.

Department of Health (2008) *End of Life Care Strategy. Promoting High Quality Care for all Adults at the End of Life*. DoH, London.

Ellershaw, J. and Wilkinson, S. (2003) *Care of the Dying. A Pathway to Excellence*. Oxford University Press, Oxford.

Help the Hospices (2007) *The End of Life Care Strategy for England. How the Government Could Change the Way We Die*. Report and summary of recommendations from the hospice movement. Help the Hospices, London.

National Council for Hospices and Specialist Palliative Care Services (2006) *Changing Gear: Guidelines for Managing the Last Days of Life*. Clinical Guidelines Working Party, December 1997 (updated 2006).

National Institute for Clinical Excellence (2004) *Improving Supportive and Palliative Care for Adults with Cancer: The Manual*. NICE, London.

 Useful websites

National Council for Palliative Care
http://www.ncpc.org.uk/

The Scottish Partnership Agency for Palliative and Cancer Care
http://www.spapcc.demon.co.uk/

✏️ Chapter links to the Nursing and Midwifery Council Standards of Conduct, Performance and Ethics for Nurses and Midwives (2008)

Section 1: Make the care of people your first concern, treating them as individuals and respecting their dignity

Treat people as individuals
- You must treat people as individuals and respect their dignity
- You must treat people kindly and considerately
- You must act as an advocate for those in your care, helping them to access relevant health and social care, information and support

Collaborate with those in your care
- You must listen to the people in your care and respond to their concerns and preferences
- You must support people in caring for themselves to improve and maintain their health
- You must recognise and respect the contribution that people make to their own care and wellbeing
- You must make arrangements to meet people's language and communication needs

Ensure you gain consent
- You must ensure that you gain consent before you begin any treatment or care
- You must respect and support people's rights to accept or decline treatment and care
- You must uphold people's rights to be fully involved in decisions about their care
- You must be aware of the legislation regarding mental capacity, ensuring that people who lack capacity remain at the centre of decision making and are fully safeguarded

Section 2: Work with others to protect and promote the health and wellbeing of those in your care, their families and carers, and the wider community

Share information with your colleagues
- You must keep your colleagues informed when you are sharing the care of others

Work effectively as part of a team
- You must consult and take advice from colleagues when appropriate
- You must make a referral to another practitioner when it is in the best interests of someone in your care

Section 3: Provide a high standard of practice and care at all times

Use the best available evidence
- You must deliver care based on the best available evidence or best practice
- You must ensure any advice you give is evidence based if you are suggesting healthcare products or services
- You must ensure that the use of complementary or alternative therapies is safe and in the best interests of those in your care

Keep your skills and knowledge up to date
- You must have the knowledge and skills for safe and effective practice when working without direct supervision
- You must recognise and work within the limits of your competence
- You must keep your knowledge and skills up to date throughout your working life
- You must take part in appropriate learning and practice activities that maintain and develop your competence and performance

Keep clear and accurate records
- You must keep clear and accurate records of the discussions you have, the assessments you make, the treatment and medicines you give and how effective these have been

☑ Self-assessment test

1. The key message emerging from government policy regarding care priorities at the end of life is:
   - A   Good palliative care is cheaper than curative care
   - B   Looking after the family is very important
   - C   Increasing the number of people dying at home
   - D   Offering greater choice and care with dignity and symptoms well managed

2. The most commonly reported physical symptoms close to death include:
   - A   Confusion, weakness, loose bowels
   - B   Dyspnoea, pain, noisy breathing

C High temperature, thirst, agitation

D Lowered consciousness, glazed eyes, high blood pressure

3. When caring for the family around the bedside of someone who is dying it is important to:

   A Tell them in detail about what is likely to happen at the moment of death

   B Give them a selection of leaflets about hospital procedures regarding the death certificate and the collection of belongings

   C Encourage them to say goodbye and allow them the time, space and privacy to do so

   D Recommend a nearby restaurant for meals if they are hungry

4. Professional priorities after the person has died include:

   A Completing all relevant paper work and making sure the GP knows of the death

   B Getting last offices completed as soon as possible to free up the bed

   C Informing the duty doctor or GP that the person has died and organising last offices for after the family has left

   D Telling the coroner – just in case a post mortem is needed

5. You are asked to organise the environment around the bedside to make it more conducive to personal care. Do you:

   A Move the bed closer to the window, clear the area of unnecessary clutter, monitor the patient's breathing

   B Lower your voice around the family as a mark of respect, continue with routine observations of temperature and pulse, call the relevant faith minister

   C Open the windows to let fresh air in and the spirit out after the person has died, put on extra blankets if the person feels cold, dim the lighting

   D Use spray deodorisers generously to mask bad odours, give full bed baths regularly, take down all infusions

CHAPTER 17

Caring for the bereaved

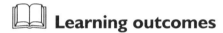 *We had been together for over forty years, Tom and I. I loved him and at times I hated him. He was my life, my love, my inspiration, my reason to be. Now he is dead. This is not how I planned it. My heart SCREAMS out with pain and every sentence begins with 'If only'.*

Learning outcomes

After reading this chapter and completing the reflective activities the learner will be able to:

■ Understand loss and grief as a normal life event
■ Describe the feelings, behaviours and thoughts experienced by those facing loss and grief and relate these to nursing practice
■ Describe a range of helping strategies that can be used to help the bereaved

Introduction

Throughout life we experience many losses and constant change. According to Littlewood (1992), a quarter of the world's population will be experiencing the death of someone close who has died in the last five years. Josef Stalin said, 'The death of one person is a tragedy, the death of a million is a statistic'. To all patients and those who love them loss is a tragedy. For staff who care for patients their death is never merely a statistic.

The latter half of the 20th century has seen death, dying and bereavement become topics that are taboo conversation in everyday life, even though they are something that everyone experiences (Johnson, 2004). This has created generations of people whose direct life experience of dealing with the loss of a loved one is limited mostly to the latter part of their life, and now in the 21st century we find ourselves more and more dependent on healthcare professionals to demonstrate and role model the behaviours and skills needed to deal with this major life event (DoH, 2008). The paradox, of course is that nurses come from the same communities as those bereaved and have been exposed to the same life-limiting sociological factors as the people they are expected to help. It is a sobering thought to be regarded by the dying and the bereaved as a role model and expert, when the reality for most nurses in clinical practice is that they often feel just as inadequate and lost for words as those around them.

There is a strong argument therefore that we have a duty to encourage discussion about such events in a way that makes them more acceptable to those we care for (Arnason & Hafsteinsson 2003). Greater awareness of these life events in a context of normality could enhance health and wellbeing and also allow people and communities to be more aware and supportive of the bereaved. It does appear, however, that dealing with loss, grief and bereavement, particularly within health and social care, is becoming increasingly challenging.

Defining loss, grief and bereavement

Clear definitions of loss, grief and bereavement are surprisingly hard to find, which is probably indicative of the vast range of authors who have attempted to analyse and explain this life event, all of whom have approached it from a different perspective. Whilst in some respects this can be seen as a good thing, as such diverse analysis can add considerably to our understanding, in the reality of everyday clinical practice it can serve to confuse rather than clarify. The definitions offered therefore have been chosen for both their inherent simplicity and timeless transparency.

Loss:
> ... deprived of, or being without, a valued someone or something one has had or ought to have... (Jacob, 1993)

Grief:

> ... a normal dynamic individualised process which pervades every aspect (physical, emotional, social and spiritual) of persons experiencing the loss... (Jacob 1993)

Bereavement:

> benefiting the bereaved individual, to help him or her to deal with the emotional and practical problems following the loss of a loved one (Schut *et al.*, 2001, p. 705).

As you can see, the Jacob definition of loss can apply to many life scenarios, from losing your car keys, through to divorce or even failing an important examination. It emphasises that loss is a common life experience that affects all of us throughout our daily lives. The grief definition also emphasises the normality of the event and that it needs to be viewed as a holistic concept that is ever changing and not as a medical condition with symptoms. Schut's bereavement definition reinforces this by stressing the notion of help offered by others and from self to deal with the emotional and practical difficulties faced day by day.

Reflective activity

When we think of loss in the context of palliative care we naturally think of death, but if you think back over your own life you will be able to think of other losses. Moving house aged 11 results in the loss of a way of life and friends. Leaving home aged 18 to start work, university or to marry results in enormous changes. Broken relationships as a result of divorce or separation, redundancy, infertility, illness and momentous world events all affect us to some extent.

Think back to some of the losses you have suffered during your life and make a list of some of the emotions you experienced.

Feedback

It is likely that you felt some of the following:

- Pain
- Anger
- Distress
- Bewilderment
- Relief
- Guilt
- Mistrust
- Emptiness
- Loneliness
- Distraught
- Confusion

Evolving perspectives on bereavement particularly in the last four decades have resulted in a move to recognise that loss through death is not something we recover from but something that we adapt to and build into our continuing lives (Stroebe and Schut, 1999). Previous research by Parkes (2001) has also demonstrated that bereavement has an impact on health and wellbeing and as such demands attention. Engagement and interest in bereavement and bereavement care should be the responsibility of all health and social care professionals and greater understanding and development of services could have significant benefit for everybody. How to achieve this, and which aspects to develop, remain unclear as there is a plethora of perspectives and services mostly provided by the charitable sector in the UK with little coordination. In addition there is a real need to assess when provision should be balanced with promotion of self-care.

For the families who encounter bereavement the moment of death and the subsequent reactions produce a wide variety of emotions: sadness; anger; separation distress; denial; loss of interest in self and social functioning; and constant replaying of events (Parkes, 1996). However, the evidence clearly shows that the presence of such strong feelings does not equate to poor outcomes for the majority of people (Stroebe *et al.*, 2005), hence the need to consider the self-care abilities of each individual who is bereaved.

Time can soften some of the emotions but sometimes a memory, a smell or a song can bring them back into sharp focus. The process of coming to terms with loss takes a long time and the journey is scattered with pitfalls. As professionals we must remember this and provide continued support where possible. The lived experience of grief is summed up eloquently by Lewis (1961, p. 60), who says:

> Grief is like a long valley, a winding valley where any bend may reveal a totally new landscape... sometimes the surprise is the opposite one: you are presented with exactly the same sort of landscape you thought you left behind miles ago.

To illustrate this here are some anecdotal comments made by the bereaved that you may have encountered.

- It's so lonely
- It hurts, a gut wrenching pain. Will it ever go away?
- He was here, always here, now I have nothing but a hollow emptiness
- Why why why? I would do anything to bring her back
- If only
- I never told him I loved him
- Life has been hard, I just want to feel whole again

Models of grief

Many models of grief exist and all add something to our understanding. Most have distinct common denominators and their purpose is to help the reader to understand the nature and complexity of loss and to offer insights into helping the bereaved. They can be categorised as phase models, the medical model, grief work models and the grief bereavement biography model. For an excellent critical review of loss models see Anstey and Lewis (2001).

Colin Murray Parkes (1996) and William Worden (2003) write about bereavement from an attachment perspective, which originated from the work of John Bowlby (1999). Tony Walter (1999), however, brought a sociological perspective on grief, whilst Margaret Stroebe and Henk Schut (1999) offer a model of loss that sees it as a dual purpose – i.e. coping with the reality of loss firstly then dealing with the issues of everyday life.

Perhaps one of the most useful models of grief in palliative care is Worden's model (Worden, 2003), which proposed four tasks of mourning the bereaved need to attend to. By focusing on tasks he sees grief as something that is active, not passive and the individual can shape their experience by attending to them:

1. Accept the reality of the loss
2. Experience and work through the pain of grief
3. Adjust to life without the deceased
4. Emotionally relocate the deceased and move on with life

By looking at these and drawing on your personal experience one can sense the enormity of these tasks when someone loses a loved one. It may be useful to think about and list the sort of things that have helped you to cope. You may have thought of the following:

- Practical help: child care, shopping
- Someone who will listen and not tell me what to do
- Someone who will let me tell my story over and over again
- My faith
- Crying
- Quiet contemplation

In addition, the suggestions in Table 17.1 are presented to help you apply Worden's model.

One other simple concept which is easily translated to clinical practice are Bowlby's (1999) principles for successful grieving. With these four statements he is indicating that in order for the resolution of what we understand as 'normal' grief, the person needs to have these core components in place. They are neither prescriptive nor follow a linear pattern, and are not dependent on culture or sociological factors.

1. Has a reasonably secure relationship with the person prior to death
2. Prompt and accurate information. Is allowed to ask questions and receive honest answers
3. Participates in family grieving, including funeral rites
4. Has the comforting presence of a parent or another adult whom he trusts and can rely on in a continuing relationship

Table 17.1 Worden's model of grief (Worden, 2003).

Worden's task	Ways of helping
Accept the reality of the loss	Talk to the bereaved. Use clear explicit language: Dead and death rather than gone or passed on. Stay with the bereaved. Speak of the dead. Repeat the bad news Listen and explain.
Experience and work through the pain of grief	Listen and help the bereaved tell their story. Acknowledge the pain, anger and distress.
Adjust to life with-out the deceased	Revisit the story. Talk about the deceased. Practical advice about work life, money, relationships. Revisit feelings. Explore fears.
Emotionally relo-cate the deceased and move on with life	Rituals, e.g. services of remembrance. Help the deceased to say goodbye and move on without forgetting the one who has died. Talk about other relationships.

Our interpretation of 'a secure relationship' does not mean that all issues with loved ones are resolved. Real life dictates that the complexity of past life experiences can create a panoply of emotions around the bedside that may never be resolved. What is meant is that however difficult the situation, the person who is soon to be bereaved needs to come to terms with the existing reality as it is so that factors such as post-bereavement guilt are minimised.

The idea of being able to ask questions and receive honest answers is at the core of good nursing practice and is strongly endorsed by the Nursing and Midwifery Council Code of Conduct (2008). This is particularly relevant where children are concerned. There is a natural propensity for all parents to want to shield a child from potential emotional hurt and therefore either to deny them access to the dying or to couch the experience in euphemisms. This can confuse children and potentially create problems for them in the future. For example, telling a child that their grandfather has gone to sleep and will now never wake up may result in that child having a disturbed sleep pattern for some time. From the child's perspective it is the simple premise that if I go to sleep tonight it's therefore possible that I may never wake up again. We have clear and compelling evidence now that children's capacity for understanding the concrete reality of permanent loss has moved down the age range in the last 50 years and that most children and young people want to talk about things that are happening in families (Brown, 2006).

The simple idea of 'participating in family grieving including funeral rites' is all about the need to say goodbye in whatever way is appropriate for the culture and family. Once again the attendance of children at such events can be helpful, but this will depend entirely on their age and the support that is available to help them deal with the situation. Ultimately it is a parental decision, but if it is clearly not appropriate for them to attend the funeral for whatever reason then some thought should be given to how this can be addressed in the home environment at a later date, with a simple ritual of some kind. For example, the planting of a tree in the garden to remember the person, or the creation of a scrap book with pictures and mementos of the person.

It is the final part of Bowlby's principles which is perhaps the most significant. There are now more single, divorced and widowed people living alone in our society than ever before (Payne and Seymour, 2008) and the number is likely to increase. We also live in an era of ever-changing family structures and demographics where the supportive key trusted adult may not be available. It is widely acknowledged that such support will help to prevent some of the documented psychological morbidity associated with bereavement (Stroebe and Stroebe, 1994).

How can we help?

As nurses, we are all likely to deal with this issue at some time in our clinical practice as well as in our own lives. However, the need for formal intervention if grief is seen as a normal process from which most people will emerge has been questioned (Raphael *et al.*, 2001). Also, evidence of the effectiveness of such interventions is relatively weak (Jordan and Neimeyer, 2003) so that even if we believe intervention is necessary, for example counselling, the effects may not be significant.

However, there will always be some bereaved individuals who do require intervention and these should not be ignored. Although imprecise, it has been estimated that between 5% and possibly up to 33% will develop pathological grief reactions (Schut and Stroebe, 2005). We now have good evidence for certain identifiable factors that lead to those who are bereaved going on to develop complicated grief and that these factors are amenable to assessment (Prigerson *et al.*, 1995). Complicated grief may of course be accompanied by other health-related problems, like anxiety and depression, that require treatment and additional care.

Ask any professional what is difficult about caring for the dying and bereaved and many will respond, 'I don't know what to say'. We must remember that nothing will 'fix' the problem or make it all better. Often we resort to the common clichés we have learned as we grew up, for example:

- He had a good innings
- At least he is not suffering any more
- At least he is not in pain
- You will find someone else
- I know how you feel
- You have still got the twins
- Time is a healer
- You just have to get on with life
- Look on the bright side

Most of these comments do not help, apart from making us think we have done something, and some of them are dismissive and patronising, reinforcing the idea that grief should just be tolerated and suffered in private. The emotional component of grief can be described in everyday life as a magician's hat of emotions, which leap out and catch us when we least expect it (Figure 17.1).

On the good days life moves along smoothly enough, but the bereaved know there is always the threat of an unexpected trigger to interrupt their daily routines. Such triggers include:

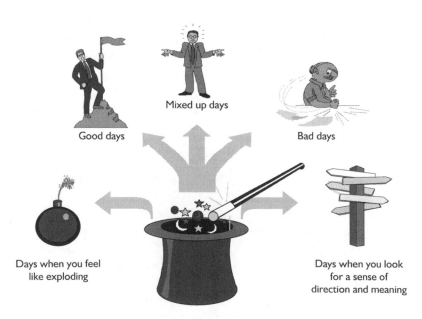

Figure 17.1 The magician's hat of emotions that accompany grief.

- **Music** – hearing a favourite tune on the radio that is associated with a particular memory of the deceased
- **Discoveries** – a photo, a piece of jewellery or a household tool or gadget. In the case of a deceased child it may be a lock of hair, a hand- or footprint or an item of baby clothing
- **Special days** – birthdays, anniversaries, Christmas, or the anniversary of the death are specially sensitive times
- **Favourite places** – countryside beauty spots that were regularly visited may hold special memories
- **People they meet** – friends relatives, strangers (even health professionals). You may be an emotional trigger for families who have had perhaps daily contact with you for some weeks and got to know you quite well
- **Habits** – familiar rituals repeated without thought, such as the laying of a place at a dining table
- **Feelings** – experiencing a feeling from an unrelated life event and then connecting it to the loss. A film on TV or a news report can be just such an event

 Reflective activity

Identify someone in your life who you know and trust who has suffered a close personal loss in the past. Ask their permission to discuss the matter, and if they agree ask them to describe the thoughts, feelings and behaviours they experienced from those around them during their grief. Ask them also to identify what helped and what hindered them. Take notes as you go along and compare these to the text in this chapter.

Feedback

Hearing the lived testimony of a person who has been through grief is the most powerful form of learning there is and can put a much clearer context to the theories and principles put forward in the literature. Hopefully you will have found some other parallels.

What can I say?

The bereaved feel even more lonely and isolated when they are ignored by family, friends and professionals. Meeting someone for the first time who is bereaved is difficult because we fear making it worse. This is very unlikely, so we must try to find words of comfort. There are no definitive answers, but the following may sometimes help.

- I don't know what to say
- I can only imagine how difficult this must be for you
- Would you like me to stay?
- I am sorry for your loss
- Would you like to talk?
- Is there anything I can do to help?
- How are you?
- How do you feel?
- Do you have any questions?

 ## Reflective activity

Take another look at the bullet list offered to you above to see if you can identify the common denominators between many of them.

Feedback

1. You may have noticed that, of the nine points, six were questions and three were statements. The questions offer the bereaved an opportunity to tell their story about their experience.
2. The three statements offered are mainly about recognising the impotence and overwhelming nature of the experience – something we can all do with care and compassion.
3. Some of the questions are open (to elicit a conversational response) and some are closed and more practical in nature. A good mix of such questions demonstrates an empathic response which is focused on helping as well as sympathy.

Myth: Many nurses fear that if they say the wrong thing then it will make the situation worse and the person may become more upset. They may then be accused of being unprofessional and lacking in competence, possibly resulting in some degree of censure.

Reality: The bereaved know that those round them find it difficult to find the right words to say and recognise that people they meet are often at a loss for the right vocabulary. Even if you fall into long-established clichés the bereaved will forgive you – as long as you demonstrate you care.

What else can I do?

Taking that first step is so important. Following up is equally important. Don't underestimate the value of making a cup of tea and sitting with the newly bereaved. You will feel you have done something and the bereaved will appreciate the kindness. The bereaved value someone who will listen and stay with them through the pain.

 Reflective activity

Case study: Josh

Read the brief background information and think about how you could offer him help and support

Josh is a 50-year-old university lecturer. He was born in Hull and moved to Edinburgh when he was 11. His grandmother died when Josh was 21 and his father died suddenly when he was 32. A very close friend moved to America 10 years ago. He separated from his wife and son 18 months ago. His mother, with whom he has always been very close, is now frail and elderly. Josh is unremarkable, yet he has suffered a number of major losses throughout his life. It is likely that he will also have experienced many other losses.

While in hospital for minor surgery you notice he is quiet and withdrawn. You ask how he is feeling and offer an opportunity to talk. He talks freely and openly about many things, including:

■ His feelings about his dad and things left unsaid
■ His marriage, his sense of failure and being judged by others
■ His feelings towards his son he misses every day
■ His fears about losing his mother in the coming years
■ His uncertainty about his future and the possibility of finding love again

After listening for a while you ask if it is possible for Josh to sum up how he feels at the moment. He talks eloquently of past pleasures and pains. 'Good friends jolly me along reassuring me that it will get better'. 'I have an overwhelming and all-consuming feeling of loneliness and missed opportunities as I struggle with each day'.

Which of the helping strategies cited above do you feel could be of most use to someone like Josh? Make a list of those you think are realistic and achievable.

Lessons learnt from the past

Grief is not a disease, and the tendency to medicalise grief, which was a feature of the narrow, process-based, linear thinking models that have pervaded the last 30 years is at last beginning to fade. The seminal work *On Death and Dying*, by Dr Elizabeth Kubler Ross (1970), which is still actively cited by many students today in grief-related essays and has provided us with a core of understanding in this area, has been superseded by a much more normalistic view. Her much-cited linear grieving process was never intended to be seen as such, and whilst it offers us an easily understood framework for the common denominators of grief in most situations, it can be argued that its misinterpretation by health professionals – nurses included – has actually added to the increasing medicalisation of grief. Even the terminology used, whilst simple and easy to understand and relate to life events, can cause confusion.

- **Denial** is a perfectly normal and acceptable mental defence mechanism which is used by all of us in daily life. In the context of grief it is also a normal reaction to an immensely stressful situation. Confusion arises because it is sometimes assumed to be an unconscious decision and the person is unaware of their action. Denial in this context is a conscious decision and is used by the person to temporarily protect themselves from the anticipated psychological pain that is imminent. It is usually transient and only ever becomes an issue when it persists over a long period of time and interferes with daily life.
- **Anger** is an emotion that none of us like to be on the receiving end of, yet is to be anticipated and expected from the recently bereaved. Anger at the health care services, anger at relatives and anger turned inwards towards self are all normal reactions. It is the potential power and unpredictability of this emotion that makes it so difficult to deal with in clinical practice.
- **Bargaining** is a poor choice of word to describe what is in fact a search for meaning to this major life event. It is well documented and understood by philosophers, theologians and health professionals that, faced with issues such as our own mortality, we feel vulnerable and need to find some sense of meaning to help us deal with the event. Whether this is through formal religious belief or other means is entirely an individual choice, but the fact remains that asking the rhetorical questions 'Why me?', 'Why this?' and 'Why now?' is common to all humanity.
- **Depression** is a clearly defined psychiatric pathology that has immense consequences for overall health and often requires a range of professional interventions to help the person recover. Whilst there is clear evidence of the associated risks for the bereaved to become clinically depressed (Stroebe *et al.*, 2005) it is by no means inevitable and can be argued that in the context of normal grief is quite rare. For this reason the use of the word 'depression' to describe normal grief is no longer appropriate. The gulf between deep-seated clinical depression and grief is enormous and its useful to look at a simple way of remembering this (see Figure 17.2).
  Think of it as three life stages:

1. For most of us life becomes emotionally difficult at times and we need to express that emotion to those close to us to help us through these times

2. The grieving person feels emotional also, but these feelings can seem take over everyday life in the short term. The intensity is more focussed. With support to enable expression this is usually worked through

3. The clinically depressed person commonly appears devoid of all emotion and needs professional psychotherapeutic intervention to facilitate expression of feelings and eventual resolution

Figure 17.2 The emotional component of grief.

1. We are at the top of the cliff with a firm hold on daily life and deal with crises as they arise.
2. We are grieving and vulnerable, but still have a firm hold on the side of the cliff. With support we can make our way back to the top.
3. The clinically depressed person is at the bottom of the cliff, with no perceived way up.

- **Acceptance** implies that there is a defined point in time when the reality of the event has become all pervading and that a person has moved on in their life and is no longer grieving. Whilst the former is true, the latter most certainly is not. The dynamic and fluid nature of grief is such that triggers and memories will occur for many years after the event and there is no defined period or time of rapid change.

Limitations to the linear concept of grief

- It should not be seen as time restricted
- The pattern of grief is often non-sequential and elements can reoccur at any time
- It should not be viewed as a checklist of medical symptomatology where any variation may be indicative of pathological grief (Walshe, 1997)
- It implies that the grieving person is a passive recipient without control over this phenomenon (Worden, 2003)
- It concentrates on the psychosocial dynamics at the expense of the physical and spiritual dimension (Farrell, 1999)

■ It implies that a valued destination and recovery is always achievable (Copp, 1998)

Risk assessment of those facing bereavement

Student nurses are inevitably close to patients and families on a physical and emotional level. They are therefore in a unique position to contribute to the assessment of bereavement risk. Carrying out bereavement risk assessment aims to reduce the long-term effects of unresolved grief and target scarce resources available to the bereaved. Factors such as age, type of death, previous bereavement experiences, social support, personal characteristics and relationship with the deceased are key criteria that may be useful in identification of those who may require additional follow up and support (Parkes, 1996). Perhaps, as nurses in all settings, we might consider how we communicate about the bereaved so that those who we identify as at higher risk can be followed up by community-based voluntary or statutory agencies. However, if services are not aware of each other or linked together in some way it may just be left to the individual to try to cope until such time as their grief presents itself in other ways (Woof and Carter, 1997)

Melliar-Smith (2002) provides a detailed account of how to perform bereavement risk assessment together with a document developed by herself and her colleagues. Consider the following aspects surrounding the illness, death and relationships between the carer and the patient:

■ Length of time patient has been in your care
■ Mode of death: sudden, peaceful or problematic
■ Main carer's understanding of illness and care
■ Spiritual and religious issues
■ Anticipatory grieving: have the patient and carers discussed death and putting affairs in order?
■ Previous life events experienced by carers: other deaths, physical or mental illness or trauma, divorce, separation, financial problems, dependent children and other relatives, employment, family conflict
■ Carer's health: physical and emotional
■ Any other issues that may affect the carer's bereavement

In general, the level of formal bereavement provision for those at risk of a complex grief reaction should depend very much on the individual, many only requiring some validation of their response and fewer requiring the use of specialised mental health and psychological services for complicated grief reactions and depression (Raphael *et al.*, 2001). Therefore we need a broad level of service to deal with the main body of bereaved and more specialised services for those who are unable to steer their own journey through grief.

Anticipatory grief

It is essential to understand that grief does not begin when the patient dies and the survivors are alone. Lindemann (1994) described grief which occurs before the death, in anticipation. The concept of anticipatory grief can be used to understand reactions leading up to death. At present there appears to be no convincing evidence that anticipatory grief work modifies the bereaved response to loss. This should not deter all staff from acknowledging losses that have and continue to occur, including approaching death.

Key nursing strategies to support the bereaved

- **By being there**: Don't attempt to offer any solutions, because there are none. In addition to practical help in the early stages, do not underestimate the value of being there and listening. Your 'presence' can be invaluable.
- **By active listening in a non-judgmental way**: Allow people time to grieve in a way that suits them. There is no right or wrong way to grieve and no predetermined time span.
- **Be clear in your intentions**: If you make a conscious decision to stay and help the person then commit yourself to this decision.
- **Accept that you cannot make them better**: This is a different kind of helping and turns the conventional concept of helping on its head. We now know quite clearly that in order for people to grieve successfully they must experience the pain that goes with it. So the job of the nurse is to be a facilitator for the expression of grief, not to deny it and attempt to heal it in some way. This is one of the few times when the often used expression 'there's no gain without pain' can be cited with accuracy.
- **Allow sadness**: Take their feelings and fears seriously and reinforce to them the normality of their experiences.
- **Expect anger**: This is a normal reaction and should not be taken personally. They may be angry with you, the doctors, god or even the person who has died.

- **Encourage them to talk of the deceased**: Ask about their life together and look at mementos and photographs. Allow them to tell their story as they see it.
- **Allow repetition**: This is very common and is known to be helpful. It helps the bereaved to make sense of what has happened.
- **Mention the deceased by name**: This helps to affirm your interest and encourages expression. 'I enjoyed caring for Bill and hearing him talk of his love for you'. Perhaps surprisingly, many family and friends avoid mentioning the deceased by name in conversation for fear of causing more emotional upset. In reality this is one of the simplest, most effective and supportive things we can do.
- **Appropriate physical contact**: Use touch in a caring sensitive way if you feel it is the right thing to do. Perhaps the most neutral place to instigate caring touch is on the outside of the upper arm, where there is little fear of misinterpretation. If the person makes it clear that they do not want such contact this will be evident to you very quickly and you can move the conversation on. It is equally true, however, that many nurses have avoided such overt demonstrations of caring even when they felt it would be helpful due to an irrational fear of assault and litigation promoted by the popular media. Context is everything, and careful judgement of the situation will rarely be shown to be wrong.
- **Tolerate silences**: People can do a lot of useful thinking in silent moments. Resist the urge to speak. This is a learned skill which is much undervalued, but takes time to develop. The next time you find yourself in such a situation, practice staying silent for up to a minute longer than you normally would. You may be surprised at the difference this makes.
- **Develop hope**: Reassure the person that difficult feelings are part of grief and that it is normal and self-limiting. Many people can feel overwhelmed by the intensity of emotions that may never have been experienced before and feel that their sanity is in danger.
- **Encourage visits** to the cemetery or the spot where the ashes may have been scattered.
- **Use treasured objects** to make links and encourage dialogue. We all have photos and mementos that can help with this.
- **Creative writing, painting and drawing** can help expression when words are difficult.
- **Writing a letter** to the deceased. Many adults and children in particular can find it easier to express themselves on paper rather than verbally. A letter takes times and can be edited until it reflects exactly what the person wants to say.
- **Encourage social contacts**. This will come slowly, but is an important part of re-establishing a normal life routine.
- **Help them to remove** emotionally painful objects to another temporary location. There can be a tendency towards emptying a house of all posses-

sions as quickly as possible because it is painful to go through the process of sorting items. Many things can therefore be lost to the charity shop or the recycling centre and the choice to retrieve it at a later date is gone.

- **Rally help from friends**, particularly close to birthdays and anniversaries and in the 6–12 week period after bereavement. It is well known that this period is often the worst for many, as family and friends who may have offered good consistent support in the first few weeks will have gone back to their lives and routines. The bereaved are then left feeling alone and isolated for the first time.
- **Be familiar with your own feelings in this area**: You need to have thought through your own reactions to death and dying in particular with past events and scars. The ability do this relates directly to the development of a mature, reflective and self-aware professional who is able to contemplate such issues and deliver nursing care of a consistently high calibre and not burn themselves out due to the inherent emotional stresses of such work.

Conclusion

Nurses in all care environments where people die will have contact with the bereaved at some point. Whilst many of these interactions will be transient, because of the nature of the clinical work, there will also be many instances where regular contact is maintained and a trusting relationship is built over time. Nurses are therefore in a key position to facilitate the expression of grief and support the bereaved in many circumstances ranging from the resuscitation room in an emergency department through to the side room of a local hospice. The skills involved are not specialist in nature; they cross all branches of nursing and the evidence base in support of nurses' involvement and success in such care is compelling. It requires a confident, mature and self-assured practitioner to stay with the bereaved in difficult circumstances, but the rewards are immense and it is without doubt one of the most challenging but satisfying areas nursing practice.

References

Anstey, S. and Lewis, M. (2001) Bereavement, grief and mourning. In: *Palliative Nursing: Bringing Comfort and Hope* (eds. S. Kinghorn and R. Gamlin). Baillière Tindall, Edinburgh.

Arnason, A. and& Hafsteinsson, S. B. (2003) The revival of death: expression, expertise and governmentality. *British Journal of Sociology*, **54**(1), 43–62.

Bowlby, J. (1999) *The Making and Breaking of Affectional Bonds*. Basic Books, London.

Brown, J. (2006) Young people and bereavement counselling. What influences their decision to access professional help? *Bereavement Care*, **25**(1), 3–6.

Copp, G. (1998) A review of current theories of death and dying. *Journal of Advanced Nursing*, **28**(2), 382–90.

Department of Health (2008) *End of Life Care Strategy. Promoting High Quality Care for all Adults at the End of Life*. DoH, London.

Farrell, P. (1999) The limitations of current theories of understanding bereavement and grief. *Counselling*, May, 143–6.

Jacob, S. (1993) An analysis of the concept of grief. *Journal of Advanced Nursing*, **18**, 1787–94.

Johnson, K. (2004) Grief in North America, a death denying society. *International Journal of Palliative Nursing*, **10**(9), 435.

Jordan, R. and Neimeyer, R. A. (2003) Does grief counselling work? *Death Studies*, **27**(9), 765–86.

Kubler Ross, E. (1970) *On Death and Dying*. Tavistock, London.

Lewis, C. S. (1961) *A Grief Observed*. London.

Lindemann, E. (1994) Symptomatology and the management of acute grief. *American Journal of Psychiatry*, **101**, 141–8.

Littlewood, J. (1992) *Aspects of Grief: Bereavement in Adult Life*. London, Routledge.

Melliar-Smith, C. (2002) The risk assessment of bereavement in a palliative care setting. *International Journal of Palliative Nursing*, **8**(6), 281–7.

Parkes, C. M. (1996) *Bereavement: Studies of Grief in Adult Life*, 3rd edn. Routledge, London.

Parkes, C. M. (2001) A historical overview of the scientific study of bereavement. In: *Handbook of Bereavement Research: Consequences, Coping and Care* (eds. M. S. Stroebe *et al.*). American Psychological Association, Washington.

Payne, S. and Seymour, J. (2008) Chapter 1, p. 30 in: *Palliative Care Nursing: Principles and Evidence for Practice* (eds. S. Payne, J. Seymour and C. Ingleton). McGraw-Hill, Open University Press, London.

Prigerson, H. G., Maciejewski, P. K., Reynolds, C. F., Bierhals, A. J., Newson. J. T., Fasiczka, A., Frank, E., Doman, J. and Miller, M. (1995) Inventory of Complicated Grief: a scale to measure maladaptive symptoms of loss. *Psychiatry Research*, **59**(1), 65–79.

Raphael, B., Minkov, C. and Dobson, M. (2001). Psychotherapeutic and pharmacological intervention for bereaved persons. In: *The Handbook of Bereavement Research: Consequences, Coping and Care* (eds. M. S. Stroebe *et al.*). American Psychological Association, Washington.

Schut, H. and Stroebe, M. S. (2005) Interventions to enhance adaptation to bereavement. *Journal of Palliative Medicine*, **8**(suppl. 1), S140–7.

Schut, H., Stroebe, M. S., Van den Bout, J. and Terheggen, M. (2001) The efficacy of bereavement interventions: determining who benefits. In: *Handbook of Bereave-*

ment Research: Consequences, Coping and Care (eds. M. S. Stroebe *et al*.). American Psychological Association, Washington.

Stroebe, M. and Stroebe, W. (1994) The mortality of bereavement. In: *Handbook of Bereavement* (eds. M. Stroebe, W. Stroebe and R. O. Hanson). Cambridge University Press, Cambridge.

Stroebe, M. S. and Schut, H. (1999) The dual process model of coping with bereavement: rationale and description. *Death Studies*, **23**, 197–224.

Stroebe, W., Schut, H. and Stroebe, M. S. (2005) Grief work, disclosure and counselling: do they help the bereaved? *Clinical Psychology Review*, **25**, 395–414.

Walshe, C. (1997) Whom to help? An exploration of the assessment of grief. *International Journal of Palliative Nursing*, **3**(3), 132–7.

Walter, T. (1999) *On Bereavement*. Open University Press, Buckinghamshire.

Woof, W. R. and Carter, Y. H. (1997) The grieving adult and the general practitioner: a literature review in two parts (Part 2). *British Journal of General Practice*, **47**(421), 509–14.

Worden, W. J. (2003) *Grief Counselling and Grief Therapy: A Handbook for the Mental Health Practitioner*, 3rd edn. Routledge, London.

Web sites and organisations that offer support to the bereaved

Child Death Helpline
Bereavement Services Dept, Great Ormond Street Hospital, Great Ormond Street, London WC1N 3JH
http://www.childdeathhelpline.org/
Telephone: 0800 282986

Childhood Bereavement Network
Huntingdon House, 278–290 Huntingdon Street, Nottingham NG1 3LY
http://www.ncb.org.uk/
Telephone: 0115 9118070

Cruse Bereavement Care
Cruse House, 126 Sheen Rd, Richmond, Surrey TW9 1UR
http://www.crusebereavement.org.uk/
Telephone: 0208 9399530

Compassionate Friends
53 North Street, Bristol BS3 1EN
http://www.tcf.org.uk/
Telephone: 0117 966 5202

Samaritans
http://www.samaritans.org.uk/
Telephone: 01753 531011 (Local branches in telephone directory)

Winston's Wish
http://www.winstonswish.org.uk/
Telephone: 0845 2030405

Chapter links to the Nursing and Midwifery Council Standards of Conduct, Performance and Ethics for Nurses and Midwives (2008)

Section 1: Make the care of people your first concern, treating them as individuals and respecting their dignity

Treat people as individuals
- You must treat people as individuals and respect their dignity
- You must treat people kindly and considerately
- You must act as an advocate for those in your care, helping them to access relevant health and social care, information and support

Respect people's confidentiality
- You must respect people's right to confidentiality
- You must ensure people are informed about how and why information is shared by those who will be providing their care
- You must disclose information if you believe someone may be at risk of harm, in line with the law of the country in which you are practising

Collaborate with those in your care
- You must listen to the people in your care and respond to their concerns and preferences
- You must support people in caring for themselves to improve and maintain their health
- You must recognise and respect the contribution that people make to their own care and wellbeing
- You must make arrangements to meet people's language and communication needs
- You must share with people, in a way they can understand, the information they want or need to know about their health

Section 2: Work with others to protect and promote the health and wellbeing of those in your care, their families and carers, and the wider community

Share information with your colleagues
- You must keep your colleagues informed when you are sharing the care of others

Work effectively as part of a team
- You must consult and take advice from colleagues when appropriate
- You must make a referral to another practitioner when it is in the best interests of someone in your care

Section 3: Provide a high standard of practice and care at all times

Use the best available evidence
- You must deliver care based on the best available evidence or best practice

Keep your skills and knowledge up to date
- You must have the knowledge and skills for safe and effective practice when working without direct supervision
- You must recognise and work within the limits of your competence
- You must take part in appropriate learning and practice activities that maintain and develop your competence and performance

☑ Self-assessment test

1. You're visiting a patient with a district nurse and it emerges in conversation that her husband died only four weeks ago. She is complaining of not sleeping well, a poor appetite and of sometimes thinking that she hears his voice around the house. This is consistent with:
   A A depressive illness
   B Complex unresolved grief
   C A normal grief reaction
   D A psychotic illness

2. Denial:
   A Must always be challenged, because it can cause problems
   B Is a normal mental defence mechanism
   C Can be reduced by the prescription of antidepressants
   D Always resolves itself in time

3. Models of grief can offer us:
   A   A framework for understanding a persons reaction to loss
   B   A means by which we can track the symptoms of grief and anticipate patterns of behaviour
   C   A linear time-related scale of what will happen
   D   An academic means of analysis

4. Most nurses fear dealing with a grieving patient and family because they find it difficult to know what to say, so avoid the situation where possible. Which ONE of the following is correct with regard to this statement?
   A   It is true
   B   It is false
   C   It depends on the confidence and maturity of the nurse
   D   It's only possible to do this well if you have attended a course on the subject

5. Some of the strategies that can be used to help the bereaved include:
   A   Accept that you can't make things better, tell them to visit their GP and to get on with their life
   B   Encourage expression of fears and worries, active listening, recognising the importance of letting them tell their story
   C   Give them time to themselves, tell the person that grief will resolve itself in about 6 months, draw on the family for support
   D   Become a bereavement counsellor, know when to refer them on to more specialist services, tell them to visit the grave

Self-assessment test answers

Part 1: Core concepts and developments

Chapter 1: What is palliative nursing?
1. C
2. B
3. B
4. D
5. A

Chapter 2: Palliative nursing skills: what are they?
1. D
2. C
3. C
4. False
5. D

Chapter 3: Care pathways
1. D
2. B
3. C
4. A
5. B

Chapter 4: Palliative care for all diagnoses
1. B
2. C
3. A
4. D
5. D

Chapter 5: Dealing with ethical dilemmas
1. C
2. B
3. B
4. D
5. C

Part 2: Delivering hands-on care

Chapter 6: Encountering death for the first time
1. B
2. C
3. D
4. False
5. True

Chapter 7: Communicating with care and compassion
1. C
2. D
3. B
4. C
5. D

Chapter 8: The nature of pain and suffering
1. B
2. B
3. A
4. B
5. B

Chapter 9: The assessment of pain
1. A
2. A
3. C
4. D
5. C

Chapter 10: The management of pain
1. C
2. C
3. A

4. C
5. B
6. B
7. D
8. C
9. B
10. B
11. C
12. D
13. A
14. B
15. D

Chapter 11: Managing symptoms other than pain
1. C
2. B
3. C
4. D
5. D

Chapter 12: Spiritual care
1. B
2. A
3. C
4. D
5. C

Chapter 13: Palliative care emergencies
1. D
2. A
3. D
4. C
5. B

Part 3: Life closure skills

Chapter 14: Essential comfort measures at the bedside
1. C
2. A
3. D
4. B
5. C

Chapter 15: Multicultural needs at the end of life
1. C
2. B
3. A
4. D
5. B

Chapter 16: Care priorities in the last days of life
1. D
2. B
3. C
4. C
5. A

Chapter 17: Caring for the bereaved
1. C
2. A
3. A
4. C
5. C

Answers to palliative care quiz

		True	False
1.	Palliative care is only appropriate in situations where there is evidence of a downhill trajectory or deterioration		✓
2.	In palliative care, dying is seen as a normal life event	✓	
3.	The practice of palliative care is compatible with aggressive curative treatment		✓
4.	The extent of the disease determines the method of pain treatment		✓
5.	To palliate means to relieve symptoms by the use of pharmacology		✓
6.	Hospice care is a concept and philosophy rather than a building	✓	
7.	Given the choice most people would wish to die in a hospital setting		✓
8.	Competency assessment tools are an objective measure of job performance		✓
9.	Life closure skills, psychosocial care and teamwork are core areas of competency for nurses using the palliative approach	✓	
10.	People dying in hospitals feel lonely and isolated from those around them	✓	
11.	The provision of palliative care services requires emotional detachment		✓
12.	When encountering death for the first time it is useful to open the window afterwards to release the person's spirit and to bring fresh air around the bedside		✓
13.	Patient choice in how and where people die can be enhanced by the use of care pathways	✓	
14.	The Liverpool Care Pathway and Gold Standards Framework have the potential to transform palliative care in the UK	✓	
15.	Drug addiction is a major problem when morphine is used on a long-term basis for the management of pain		✓
16.	Artificial hydration at the end of life can cause the patient more harm than good	✓	
17.	Advance directives (living wills) now have full legal status in the UK	✓	
18.	During the terminal stages of an illness, drugs that can cause respiratory depression are appropriate for the treatment of severe dyspnoea	✓	
19.	Individuals who are taking opioids should also follow a bowel regime	✓	

	True	False
20. Suffering and physical pain are synonymous		✓
21. Adjuvant therapies are important in managing pain	✓	
22. The use of placebos is appropriate in the treatment of some types of pain		✓
23. In high doses, codeine causes more nausea and vomiting than morphine	✓	
24. Morphine is the standard used to compare the analgesic effect of other opioids	✓	
25. Managing symptoms other than pain is mostly about finding the right drug and dosage		✓
26. The pain threshold is lowered by anxiety or fatigue	✓	
27. Manifestations of chronic pain are different to those of acute pain	✓	
28. Pethidine is not an effective analgesic for the control of chronic pain	✓	
29. Dyspnoea, nausea and constipation are the three most common symptoms reported after pain	✓	
30. The very idea of an emergency in palliative care is a contradiction in itself		✓
31. Hypercalcaemia can be life threatening if not treated promptly	✓	
32. Spinal cord compression appears rapidly and can resolve itself spontaneously		✓
33. Telling the patient the truth about their illness if they request it is likely to cause them harm		✓
34. It's always a good idea when handling sensitive questions to seek more information first from the patient	✓	
35. Silences are difficult and are best handled by using open questioning		✓
36. The families feelings about the patient knowing their prognosis are always secondary to the patient's wishes	✓	
37. Spiritual care is best delivered by those who know most about it, i.e. ministers of a faith		✓
38. Agnostics, atheists and humanists are people who can't make their mind up what they believe		✓
39. If nurses are trained better to deliver spiritual care then it would make a big difference to the patients		✓
40. Essential comfort care around the bedside of the dying are mostly routine functional tasks that are better suited to a healthcare assistants role		✓
41. Last offices is a routine procedure that is best learnt from a policy manual		✓
42. During the last days of life, drowsiness associated with electrolyte imbalance may decrease the need for sedation	✓	

	True	False
43. It is crucial for family members to remain at the bedside until death occurs		✓
44. Cheyne–Stokes breathing is when the dying person's respiration becomes intermittent	✓	
45. Natural light and normal conversation around the bedside of a dying person can help both patient and family	✓	
46. Cultural care is full of sensitive pitfalls and it's best to call in faith leaders and let them deal with it		✓
47. Truth telling regarding diagnosis and prognosis varies in acceptability in some cultures	✓	
48. Men generally reconcile their grief more quickly than women		✓
49. The loss of a distant contentious relationship is easier to resolve than one that is close or intimate		✓
50. Grief can best be described as a time-limiting process occurring through specific stages		✓

Index